BRAINSTORM

BRAINSTORM

A Memoir of Love, Devotion, and a Cerebral Aneurysm

Robert Wintner

YUCCA

Yucca Publishing books may be purchased in bulk at special discounts for sales promotion, corporate gifts, fund-raising, or educational purposes. Special editions can also be created to specifications. For details, contact the Special Sales Department, Yucca Publishing, 307 West 36th Street, 11th Floor, New York, NY 10018 or yucca@skyhorsepublishing.com.

Yucca Publishing® is an imprint of Skyhorse Publishing, Inc.®, a Delaware corporation.

Visit our website at www.yuccapub.com.

10 9 8 7 6 5 4 3 2 1

Library of Congress Cataloging-in-Publication Data is available on file.

Cover design by Yucca Publishing

Print ISBN: 978-1-63158-020-8
Ebook ISBN: 978-1-63158-024-6

Printed in the United States of America

For Carol Kato, who often sees the picture

CONTENTS

Author's Note   IX
Prologue: Comfort Can Fool You   XI

1   Before Love Came to Town   01

2   Happily Ever After   15

3   Will You Get Away From Me? Just Get the Fuck Away!   23

4   Doogie Howser   41

5   An Exercise in Faith   53

6   You're Doing So Many Things to Upset Us   75

7   The Gift of the Ages   105

8   The Angels Sing   121

9   Time for Service!   135

10 Stuck in the Valley   155

11 Free at Last   171

Author's Note

A trepan is a hole saw, and trepanation is the process of making a burr hole in the skull to treat disease or relieve pressure. Evidence of trepanation occurs through the ages, back to Neolithic times, as a likely remedy for epilepsy, migraines and mental disorders.

Dutch painter Hieronymus Bosch depicted trepanation in his painting *The Extraction of the Stone of Madness* in about 1500, showing a patient sitting clothed in a chair as the physician operates.

Nautical author Patrick O'Brian had Dr. Stephen Maturin, particular friend of Captain Jack Aubrey (the *Master and Commander* series), perform the procedure on deck in similar fashion. Today's craniotomy is similar, though significantly sanitized.

The American Medical Association estimates about 3% of the general population to have cerebral aneurysm that may or may not leak (hemorrhage). The age group at highest risk is forty to forty-nine. Fifty to fifty-nine is second highest risk. Sixty and over is relatively low risk. This narrative is based on actual events. The names have been changed to discourage the litigants.

—RW

Prologue

Comfort Can Fool You

I see people walking down the street, talking on cell phones, or standing in doorways, talking to themselves. They reflect a mirror universe, where others are listening, and it feels like we function as a collective community, on both sides of the reflective surface. But mirror universe imagery complicates a simple idea; these people mumbling at cell phones and themselves are connected only to more of the same.

Some people pre-empt the suburban noise pattern with electronic devices clipped to their belts or strapped to their biceps, with wires dangling from tiny earphones. I feel alien and alone in an overbuilt, disconnected world. Even a beer tastes bitter, perhaps fouled by the TV overhead, where a woman bemoans "the mental welfare of our children." Mentally and physically deficient, she says, today's kids melt down in the formative years, one hour to the next in electronic interplay. This growing, obsessive pastime among the children might ensure a good supply of pilots for flight simulation, but these kids pant too easily and can't form a sentence without stumbling. They've plugged themselves in like lamps, but the bulb is dim.

I want this TV off, so I can drink my beer in solace, but the bartender is gone. Rachel should have called if she was running late. I always call her if I'm running late. So I ring her up.

"Hello."

"Where are you?"

"I . . . coming," she says, cell-phone fuzzy.

"Tonight?"

"Yeah. I . . . coming."

Oh, boy, I hear the slosh. "Look, I'll just—"

"I'm coming now." She hangs up. I wouldn't mind this pub if I could get another beer. How often do I relax like this? I think they have bars like this in hell, with overbearing TVs and you can't get served. How about a sports bar in hell where you can't get served with nothing on but golf? Where it smells like old grease and rancid bar snacks, and mortal sinners eternally suffer a guy three seats down in a tiny headset listening to the Beatles' version of *Twist and Shout*, with the music blaring loud enough from the little earplugs to compete with the overhead TV.

How can his brain withstand the sonic boom? He probably doesn't know that the Beatles did *Twist and Shout* second-hand, after the Isley Brothers did it first, nor is he likely to care. He probably thinks Aretha Franklin was first with *Respect*; he may not even know Otis Redding, much less the original *Respect*. The originals seem better, purer and closer to the source. But I also think that harking back to the olden days may indicate premature-codger syndrome. Or maybe it's time. I think the Isleys and Otis harked back bitterly, and so did Little Richard when Pat Boone poured marshmallow topping all over *Tutti Fruity*. I think Gladys Knight and the Pips got marginalized on *Heard It Through the Grapevine*, but the kids went gaga for Marvin Gaye because he had better promo. Well, at least I'm not all that bitter.

But I sense a collective consciousness verging precipitously on group mentality. Our social standards appear to be scrubbed daily by the overhead TVs of the world; reality alters as a function of ratings. Ratings are bought with huge ad budgets by media conglomerates that own the "artistic" material. It's all fair and balanced with an appropriate disclaimer. Enough people watching a thing proves the validity of the thing, just as a double-blind experiment proves a theory, kind of, and presto, a market is made. Homogenized airwaves make the world safe for those truths deemed self-evident by the largest advertisers.

I reach over the bar for the remote and surf to CNN, where a woman says flooding in Mozambique has caused gross human casualty. She is distraught and makes no mention of the clear-cutting that caused these floods, nor does she estimate prospects for watershed rejuvenation or reef recovery. Some of those humans could have been friends of mine in other circumstances, but I do believe the world will require misfortune in gradually building waves, so that the little light might shine again. What a relief to Mozambique, now that the worst is over.

Next comes Burger King on a blues riff, Toyotas with funk and soul and the show biz segment, reporting on bottom-line gross revenues on what defines our culture in Hollywood terms. The fellow down the bar shakes his head and warbles in a falsetto, "Wooo!" He grins for the boogie muse and me. I don't think the Isleys or Otis or Gladys Knight or the Pips or Little Richard would care if this guy never heard of them. Maybe they stayed happy in their art, which was different then, more a part of their lives and a reflection of their souls, as the soul genre implied, rather than a computed calculation of notes and lyrics to maximize market yield. I tell the guy down the bar, "The Isleys did it better."

"What?" He mouths the question. I shake my head. Never mind. Then again, the Isley guys did *Long Tall Sally* and *Stagger Lee*, neither one original for them. It was. . . . I don't know. Who did those, *Long Tall Sally* and *Stagger Lee?* Well, maybe I'm altogether wrong.

On the TV overhead a man in a pastel suit sincerely assures that no one should accept erectile dysfunction. The fellow three seats down pulls his plugs. "What?"

"The Isleys did it better."

"Want another?" The bartender asks on returning.

I smile and walk out. My ride is here.

Rachel might be drunk, but she smiles brightly. She often calls us the odd couple; she's so tolerant and understanding.

1

Before Love Came to Town

We met at the dog pound on Maui, Rachel and I, on a warm, sunny day. With my new house finally finished, the debris hauled off and the grass cut, a dog or two seemed in order. After all, it was a farm in the tropics; it needed some good dogs. I had many things to do that day, but then coming around the last curve out of town on the way home, the dog pound stood out like an idea with right timing. If not now, when? On impulse I pulled in.

Two women worked the place with oddly differing airs about them. The front counter woman had enhanced her womanly wares till they resounded with sexuality, visibility, cleavability, availability and, just like two rolls of plump, fresh Charmin, squeezability. Of course I dasn't, but the presentation was compelling, immobilizing me in the decision-making process. But I did decide in a blink, after all, because a man knows that a stupendous rack will not endure like true love. But I get ahead of myself; love was not yet on the table. I savored the dazzling display like a chocoholic scanning a sampler, wondering what would be better, the creamy nougat center or the crushed nuts.

Supremely suggestive, her form-fit denim presented a leggy foundation on a perfect ass with excellent lift and spread, leading up to an incredible front framed in lace and loosely covered by a man's shirt tied at the waist but straining at the braces and yearning to be free. I could have pulled the slipknot one-handed. But she glared as if at a man-dog in need of a muzzle. That glare also felt practiced and formidable. I wasn't her type. Or maybe she wanted a pursuit. Her lustrous dark hair starkly contrasted with her pale, chiseled face, like the frustrated queen in Snow White. She knew that any mirror would tell her what all men have in mind. Her waist was narrow as the evil queen's, her curvature more inspirational, beyond Disney into Crumb. I asked how things were going today at the dog pound.

"This isn't a dog pound!" she said. "We don't like that kind of talk. It's an animal shelter."

"My mistake." She returned to her work, ignoring me.

She was not Rachel. But there on the steps to the side stood a woman of more soothing profile, who was. Her natural features allured like an oasis on a tundra. She asked, "Are you looking for a companion today?" Long blonde hair framed her sparkling green eyes.

"Yes. I am." She brightened, assuring me that we could get through this with patience and understanding, and then everyone would be better off, especially the lucky pooch. "Two companions, in fact. Dogs. I have a cat."

"Two dogs? You want two?"

"I travel sometimes. They're not like cats, you know. They get depressed. If I have two, they can keep each other company when I'm gone. Can't they?"

"Well. Yes. Maybe you could get one today and see how that works out."

"Nah. I'm busy. And I'm good with dogs and cats. Don't worry. I spoil 'em rotten. I treat them like people. Well, better, actually." She smiled at my sophistry and led the way. I thought I'd done well. She told me for years afterward that I made a bigger impression than any man at the dog pound in a long time, because I wanted two. She knew then that I was special. What a woman. She showed me the old dogs, the young and middle-aged dogs. I picked two and took them home.

She seemed nice enough but hardly for me; too nice and conventional in a married sort of way. Her subtle anxiety may have been nothing but high energy, but it still felt contagious and different from my usual composure. She infused the scene with tension, like it was a pictorial from *House and Garden*, with chitchat and niceties between a single-minded bachelor and a woman wallowing in disappointment. It wasn't for me. Neither was the hard body up front, who seemed more like a centerfold from *Soldier of Fortune*.

A month later we met by chance in the grocery, Rachel and I. We recognized each other immediately, and she asked how the dogs were doing. They were doing fine, naturally. We talked dogs for a while, until I thought, singularly, why not? So I asked, "Hey. Do you want to get together for a bottle of wine?"

"A bottle?" Maybe I pressed, but I wanted to drink a bottle of wine with her so we could get decently buzzed and then screw. Is that unreasonable? No, but she faltered.

So I said, "Next week, maybe. I'll talk to you then." It seemed perfunctory and dismissive, like it would never happen. But then it did, the puzzle parts sliding into place when least expected.

For starters, she was married—not truly married but legally married, not yet divorced. I read her well enough; her guileless uncertainty gave her away. Then again, she likely read me too and wanted some wiggle room in proximity to the wolverine hunger before her. She looked away and blushed with her own mumble that maybe, I suppose, sometime, I guess, sure. I let it go. If she knocked on my door I'd offer the wine.

Another two weeks went by till I rang her up one empty afternoon to see if she wanted to take in an early movie. Well, I guess, okay, she said. I don't know why people go to movies on dates when all you do is sit in the dark for two hours beside someone you don't know any better when the credits come up. I took her home, her home, and pulled up so she could get out, because I knew she wouldn't come home with me, not on a first date. She was too classy, with a dress and lipstick and shoes and a cashmere sweater. Besides, I was too tired for the talking and feigned interest and more drinks way past cocktail hour. So I said good night; I had a great time and maybe again soon or something or other. She agreed and leaned over like it was 1962, and we kissed for a few seconds there on the front seat, and my skin went tight and my pulse kicked up, and I wondered where the hell that came from.

We went out the following week to dinner. She wore another dress, a warm-weather number in red-orange with shoulder straps and snug hips. Afterward, outside the restaurant, we stood talking to a parrot on a perch. Her thigh brushed mine, and it happened again, the electricity out of nowhere. We didn't screw for another two months simply because I knew she wouldn't. Her? Screw me? Get outta here. But then of course we did, because you must, unless you're in a monastery, where it can often take longer.

She didn't come out and tell me she was married, but I knew it from the real house and real furniture and grown-up things and the way she prepared dinner and her presentation of everything. She reeked of stability then stumbled with its opposite. Her marriage had failed but not her faith in all good things. Still she saw herself as a woman whose marriage had failed and lugged that baggage with guilt, compensating for her deficiencies, as if they were proven and must be balanced. She loved her job at the dog pound more than anything she'd ever done, because she could save cats and dogs daily by simply taking the time to find an owner or a new home for another soul so eminently adoptable. I sensed that the dogs and cats were a blessed object of her giving, her penance. I came to learn that the giving would remain compulsive, part of her character. Beyond that, the animals returned her love, which she'd been a long time without.

She rarely failed the cats and dogs and broke the rules on maximum stay at the dog pound, many times drawing the line against the time that those animals most lovable would have been led down the one-way hall to the long sleep. She would not allow them to be put down. When the kennels overflowed, she brought them home, sometimes three or five of them, old or young ones or any who asked for a break, just this once. She got them out of the pound to gain more time to find them homes. But her halfway house efforts went past compensation for anything and required no return; this was pure love. In the meantime the orphans she brought home got along more or less with her three dogs. The problem, she confided, was that she could not stay on at the dog pound indefinitely, because of the shortfall, about a grand a month between expenses and income. We had popcorn and beer in her kitchen on another evening a few months into our liaison. She seemed pleased that I took the time and effort to come over, and she didn't mind that it was ten-fifteen, after Aikido class, which had been my libido transfer for years. Now I got to transfer and eat it too, with popcorn and beer.

I remember that particular evening, because she revealed doubts on the future. I admired her by then, because many residents in a resort community wait tables or clean rooms or bell hop or sell real estate or otherwise serve the guests. No matter how much you might appreciate good service, none of it warms the heart and soul like service to the animals. Here was a woman worth pondering; saving those I loved the most.

Our dialogue then was like that first kiss. I stood back, out-of-body as it were, scenes of naked abandon only minutes away in my mind, and I heard myself say, "Yes, well, don't you worry. Now you have me to take care of you." I won't call it a psychedelic experience, but I watched the words flow out as if spoken by another self. I didn't believe them, didn't want to take care of her or anyone. I wanted sex and fun. Caring for another seemed marginally possible but hardly likely for me. Still, it seemed the thing to say because she was, after all, quite a date.

Such base assessment may seem harsh, but the truth often is, and I don't recall these drives—the lust and the nurture—as opposing. What romp is ever better than with one who cares? I have nice manners when I'm not hostile. Nor do I judge myself or seek judgment. I record what happened to more clearly understand what happened next. Which wasn't much, except for the romps and more fun than most people could ever anticipate. We went to Thailand and Malaysia, Mexico and Europe, San Francisco and Seattle. We rode the train to Vancouver and smoked hash in Amsterdam and rode another train through the Alps and walked past Chris Columbus's house in Genoa. We hiked fifteen miles across the volcanic crater at the top of Haleakala and slept there under the stars with a decent zinfandel.

We camped in the wilderness by a trout stream in Idaho. We went to the beach at Hookipa near home late afternoon on Sunday when the crowd goes away. We watched sunset, smoked a joint, drank more beer and built a fire in a ring of stones. Around the coals we set corn and potatoes wrapped in foil, and we grilled fish along with sliced egg-plant that had been soaked in olive oil. We watched the big yellow moon rise and screwed in the sand and then cleared out for home in time for Masterpiece Theater.

Like icing on cake she shared my love for the little fish of garish color and keen curiosity, and she swam like one, graceful in free dive as a dancer. She could get thirty feet and cruise for a minute on a single breath. We snorkeled many reefs in Hawaii and a dozen more in the Windward Islands of the Caribbean and a dozen more off Yucatan. We hiked for miles on deserted beaches stark naked and snorkeled again with our friends, the turtles and eels, the groupers and sharks. We achieved the bliss of Never Never, until four years in, when she told me one night after dinner that she got a call that day from the doctor about yesterday's mammogram. It showed three tiny dots, micro-calcifications that appeared acutely suspicious to the pathologist.

"I'm having a biopsy tomorrow, to be sure."

The biopsy was to remove a narrow slice of breast tissue for scrutiny under the microscope. The three dots warranted this further analysis. "Then you really don't know yet if they're tumors."

"No. But the pathologist thinks they're tumors."

"Why?"

"I don't know."

"Do you want me to go with you?"

"Would you?"

"Why wouldn't I?"

"You're busy."

"Busy with what?"

"Please don't do that."

"Okay. I'm going with you."

We watched TV, thinking inevitable thoughts. We turned in. We slept fitfully. We went in the next morning for the biopsy, and she slept off the anesthetic until after noon.

Rachel was then forty-one. She would proceed to show me the meaning of faith, initiative and courage disguised as good manners. But I recall a single moment on the second evening of our knowing; it was not another out-of-body expression but did again affirm what was to be, out of the blue, from the ether. On the phone with the pathologist, who confirmed that the three dots were tumors, she spoke evenly and wrote things down. I was taken by the calmness on the surface of her pond, and I knew this intrusion was ours to share. With nary a ripple she proceeded with life. I wanted to learn how she did that, and I knew that the trouble upon us would map our next trip together. The moment was a milestone. She hung up, smiled resolutely and said, "I have breast cancer."

I asked what she wanted to do. She didn't yet know. She would go along for now with the standard regimen of the diagnostic facility, keeping her appointments to discuss her "options." She wanted to see what they had to offer and was scheduled for next week in Honolulu to meet with the oncologist, who would explain and plan.

I foolishly asked, "Do you want me there?"

She wisely said, "Yes."

We sat and thought. Rachel has a college degree in nutrition. She owned a health-food restaurant once and remained intrigued by immune system support. Still, she stepped boldly where so many fear to tread.

The oncologist in Honolulu was an egregiously friendly fellow with a how-do-you-do and handshake for each of us. Then came polite questions on who is whom and who does what. Defaulting to grim resolve, he put a smiley face on a difficult situation, which seemed an attempt to frame our reality in black and white. On a legal pad he made line drawings of breasts and tumors, assuring Rachel that prospects for a complete cure were darn near a hundred percent. He spoke to her and only her. I was the boyfriend, an unrelated observer, more or less. Yet he seemed to sense more than indifference in my presence, perhaps ignoring the aggressor in the woodpile. I allowed for the possibility that he addressed only her in deference to legality, since boyfriends have no legal say in critical healthcare decisions, yet the exclusion felt obtuse. Maybe I observed too keenly. I remained silent with visible difficulty. Maybe he sensed my distrust.

"First, we'll have major mastectomy. This is standard procedure now. Many, many women are doing this with wonderful results. By removing the breast entirely, we can eliminate what you might call habitat for these tumors and any others." The happy face dissolved to scientific certainty.

"Why not remove both breasts?" I asked, perhaps challenging his case, in fact pressing for insight on the complete picture. "I mean, if habitat removal is the best course."

With a happy face again, he nodded approval. "Well, in fact, many women do have both breasts removed, to be sure." He smiled most warmly here. "Yes. We can do that. It's okay." He seemed oddly gratified that the question had been asked, and he'd had the right answer ready, apparently oblivious to my cynical sense of irony. Or maybe he chose to ignore the sarcastic side of the question. I was a subtle smart ass with chronic symptoms, to be sure, but in this case my pre-rational nuance was a source of effective realization.

Rachel and I shared the quizzical response.

"Secondly, we'll put you up for three days a week for twelve weeks at a very nice place just down the road here so you can be all comfy cozy during your radiation treatments. And I'm going to tell you right now"—he touched her gently, a smarmy, learned technique in vogue then with an obscure name, something like neuro-transmittal response. It should have been called operant conditioning with cheese—"don't you worry about a thing. This is all covered by your insurance. We'll start with small doses and then we'll build you up."

"Build her up? With radiation? Don't you mean you increase the dosage?"

"Do you mind? Can I finish here?"

"Sorry."

"Then, just to be sure, we'll have some chemotherapy. You won't feel so good during that one. Do you have someone who can take care of you?"

Well, I deserved a set-up like that. I was the fool nobody could see, and I laughed. But Rachel didn't need a pissing contest. She interjected quickly, softly and to the point. "Don't radiation and chemotherapy destroy my natural immunity?"

"No. We don't know that."

"We don't know that cigarette smoking causes lung cancer either, do we?" This widely broadcast corollary came from me, to sustain clarity on what we know of predisposition in the medical industry. I am inclined to disbelieve many if not most claims or contentions or, worst of all, mere suggestions of the medical industry, compromised and challenged as it is by the legal industry. I didn't mean to indicate that the oncologist was a chump; it just came out that way, and this exchange only heightened my prejudice.

"We need to schedule you right away, to be sure." He again ignored my foolish question and me.

"I'm not having surgery," Rachel said.

"What do you mean, you're not having surgery?"

"What part of that statement don't you understand?" I asked.

"We have trouble here," he said. "We have a young woman threatened by a fatal condition, and now she's being led astray."

"But it's not his decision, is it?" she asked.

"No, it's not!"

"It's mine, isn't it?"

"Yes, it is. And I'm behind you all the way."

"I'm not having surgery. I understand why tumors grow, I think. I think people have carcinogens passing through their bodies every day. All people do. The carcinogens take hold when the immune system can't get rid of them."

"That's right. But we can get rid of them."

"But with your way, I'll weaken my immune system for the future, won't I?"

He shook his head. "We want to give you a future."

"Won't I weaken my immune system?"

On the verge of indiscretion he glared, his head shaking slowly as a grandfather pendulum.

She proceeded. "I think I'm better off if I can *strengthen* my immune system and see if that can get rid of the tumors. That way I won't risk my life every time I travel, when I'll be exposed to simple infection. Doesn't that make sense?" His headshake continued. "Why not? You know these treatments compromise immunity. Isn't this entire condition based on the immune system?"

He fumed and reddened like a dormant volcano on the verge of awakening, and he stood. "What we have here is another tragedy in the making. What we have here is a breast-fixated man who's willing to risk the life of his . . . his . . . girlfriend for his own petty lusts."

Well, now, that was aggressive. *Another* tragedy? Had others also declined this guidance? Never mind; I also stood. "What we have here is a perfect stranger coming on warm and fuzzy with a knife and drugs and gamma rays. What we have here is presumption. You need a Q-tip so you can clean the . . . the . . . stuff outa your ears, so you can hear what this woman wants. Get the picture?"

He leaned forward, but what could he do? Take a shot? Oh, baby. His movement was mere posturing—but then so was mine, rendering a scene of two jerks sorting personal problems. By now Rachel was also up, telling me to shut up and sit down, or I wouldn't be welcome back. She turned to the indignant man in the white robe and said, "I apologize for his behavior. But he's listening to me more than you are. I'm not having surgery. That's my decision. Thank you very much." And out she stormed, leaving Dr. Strangelove and me to fume and mumble.

She just said no and kept on saying it. When the months and years passed with no recurrence, they called her a nut, a lucky nut, like she drew an ace to a king with the dealer showing twenty. That's how it is when you do something right; it looks easy.

She went to saturation-level vitamins and antioxidants. We searched for the guidance not offered by the American Medical Association.

Information other than promotional good cheer on radiation, surgery and chemotherapy was extremely hard to find in the days before the Internet. Either you knew exactly where to look, or you found yourself at the end of your line, pleading to the thin air. We contacted clinics with offices in San Diego and treatment facilities in Tijuana, because all cancer treatment not sanctioned by the AMA was illegal in the USA.

We visited John Yung, a Chinese healer in Honolulu who saved Suzie Schwab from kidney cancer after a licensed member of the AMA gave up, giving her three weeks to live, six on the outside. You will die then, she was told. It's not so bad, given the time to put your affairs in order.

Suzie and her husband Sylvan run the East Maui Animal Refuge, an otherworldly scene in which no animal is put down. Three-legged dogs, one-eyed cats, wingless ducks and chickens, homeless goats, piglets delivered from dead feral sows in the act of butchering, a blind owl and on and on. What a couple of nuts, Sylvan and Suzie. They heard about Rachel and called with information on John Yung. That's how you find out; people hear and call you, which isn't exactly underground, but then in the Age of Information, it's not exactly not.

He was seventy or eighty and put Rachel on a ten-day fast on the same regimen he'd prescribed for Suzie and all cancer patients. Rachel went from a hundred pounds to eighty-seven. She drank the juice of red potato skins, a five-pound bag's worth a day, and tied her gut in knots with raw vinegar straight up, an ounce in the morning and an ounce in the evening to change her body's pH in order to discourage the unwanted guest. Since then this approach has been poo pooed, though Rachel's effort, if anecdotal, proved successful.

Then came *noni*, a yellow fruit that grows in Hawaii on a bush-like tree. It looks like a lemon from afar but is thin-skinned like a nectarine. *Noni* gets mushy as it ripens till it turns to pure squish. Up close it will bend your knees, because it smells bad, like socks and skivvies after the game, unwashed. The old Hawaiians discovered the curative power of *noni* over their worst affliction before the missionaries, melanoma. More recent Hawaiians have applied *noni* to other forms of cancer with success.

And *noni* is now highly promoted and marketed around the world as a cure-all for what ails you. It's often mass harvested and cut with white grape juice, and like many truths and sacred treasures once held dear, it has been largely homogenized by a world of growing demand.

But I digress; in the mid-90's *noni* was still an obscure, little known plant referenced only by the culturally savvy for its use in olden times.

So there we were, a pair of oddballs by the side of the road out toward Makena, back when Makena Road was made of dirt, or Wainapanapa on the windward side, where the *noni* also grows wild. We found it, picked it, quartered it, put it in a sun tea jar with a tap and let it sit. We watched in wonder as the *noni* first changed with a brown mottling, then darkened and went cloudy and then mushy. Then it generated liquid. Rachel drew off and drank half a cup in the morning and another half in the evening. She observed that *noni* juice never fermented, indicating magic in the enzymes, the building blocks of immunity.

Then came more and more again—chaparral was favored as heavy medicine by the Indians of the southwest. Now it's illegal, banned by the FDA under pressure from the AMA. Chaparral has been proven a hundred percent effective anecdotally but has yet to yield ninety-six percent or better results in the double-blind format. Its subsequent illegality is based on its harsh astringent effect on the kidneys, and also on what Dr. Andrew Weil calls arrogance. The same goes for essiac, red clover and sassafras—yes, the same root I picked as a child for tea, the active taste in root beer—illegal. But if you take the time to seek these things, you may find them.

We dabbled in meditation, or rather she dabbled; I was a practitioner. She said she really liked it, except for the sitting still when she had so much to do. And so much not to do; she went cold turkey on fat, salt, beer, wine, liquor and caffeine. She took a year to gain her weight back because everything she ate was either raw or slightly warmed. She reluctantly agreed to attend a "cancer survivors group" at the urging of those who insisted on monitoring her deviant behavior. The cancer survivors group was mostly women and the format was like AA, with each survivor at the podium giving her name and saying, "I have cancer." Then each gave her treatment regimen, her progress along the path of that regimen, her feelings and out-look for the future.

This is called validation and derives from the psychiatric wing of the protocol section of the policy department of the AMA—or maybe that's only my take. Then the survivor shares her status on the road to recovery. None of the survivors but one had hair. All but one were ashen. One woman could hardly speak because her tongue was swollen to resemble a small salami as a result of the radiation. She said, "Ah tho ha-y. I ohy ha wuh mo raiathu tweauh. I juh wah geh ih eh ah geh ih ovah tho I cah bea ith thig." *I'm so happy. I only have one more radiation treatment. I just want to get in there and get it over so I can beat this thing.*

Rachel told them she'd had no surgery, no radiation and no chemo-therapy. She looked vital, so full of life you could only wonder what she was doing about her cancer. "I don't think I have it anymore," she told the others. But she didn't think anything had changed on its own, she said, proceeding to share her program of vitamins and exotic elixirs.

But . . . can we do this? They collectively suddenly doubted their regimens. Rachel told me later that she could see them poised on the brink of hazard. She told them, "You're all doing exactly what you should do. We all have to do what we believe is best for us." And she stepped down, assuring me that she'd felt compromised, forced to present herself and her regimen in a format that was meant to make her look reckless but actually cast doubt in the minds of the others. She would not go back.

And we moved on, measuring "survival" in six-month incre-ments, each a milestone with a mammogram showing clean, healthy tits. The attending surgeon on Maui was older and more reason-able than the consulting doctor in Honolulu. I think the difficult people of the world are destined to deal with each other, so he and I only answered our fates. The second doctor reviewed the film neg-atives, repeated the pathology assessment, copped a feel, smiled and shook his head. Oh, and he mumbled something new on each visit, like: "You're a lucky one," or, "I only hope this doesn't turn on you," or, "We can't be sure on this one," or, "Please don't give anyone else any ideas," or, "We'll really never know." He never said, "What a nut." I think he was too polite. At any rate, we all got along.

Dr. Strangelove called Rachel from Honolulu from time to time to "see how you're doing." Each time he asked if she was still hanging out with, you know, that guy. His interest was strictly professional, and so was his offer to examine her, you know, socially, should she find herself in town with a few hours to kill and some ignorance she'd like to process.

"Oh, yes. He's still around," she said every time. And, "I'll sure call you," she replied to his invitation.

But proving a point on health and healing with a few surgeons was small glory compared to the real triumph, which was rediscovering the power of nature and putting it on equal ground inside the body as well as outside. Initial perception of Rachel as "a lucky one" changed soon enough as women came to her, women who heard through the grapevine that she just said no. They came with constrained hope, these women who faced the malignant prognosis. They feared as we had feared and wanted to say no, but didn't know where to turn, unless Rachel had something to share.

She wrote her regimen down for them, eight or ten pages of it. She preferred longhand but couldn't say why. She spent hours with those who sought further guidance, maybe ten women in all, most with breast cancer and some with other tumors. I don't know if any of them could achieve what she did; I tried the vinegar once. It's not a matter of will or fortitude; the throat constricts and refuses. Difficulty with the *noni* began from five yards out. But in the face of rare achievement she remained humble, facing each mammogram with anxiety. Each one felt like another roll of the bones, and each helped insulate the raw nerve the doctors so brazenly touched. Confirmed in her choice, affirmed in her transformation, enforced in her skill, she viewed life as a manageable process no matter what, as long as you know where to get the right information and remedy. She was a winner, gold medal, center stand.

Oh, say, can you see?

2

———•◆•———

Happily Ever After

You think a story has a beginning and an end, but it doesn't. How can we live happily ever after, knowing that we die at the end? Well, we can because we make the best of a difficult situation, which is life with a few lovely passages if you're lucky. One problem resolves. Others form like thunderheads on the horizon.

We move forward a few years, moving in the meantime from Hawaii to Seattle, from dating to shacking up to marriage, moving as well through the ups and downs of happiness. We processed, as married people must do, all the niggling irritants so willfully caused by the other. Like being left to wait when she knows I'm so busy and hardly have time to waste in a decent bar much less a foul-smelling sports bar with bad service. Yet I learned long ago that dissatisfaction conveyed by facial expression is too easily ignored. You must verbalize your irritation.

"Listen. Are you listening to me?" She lolls her head my way, but who can tell if it's a perk or a flop? I think she's been drinking, and I can't tell if she's listening. She can piss me off, but I also learned long ago to get unpissed at the end of the day—better to relax and ease on into the evening. So I keep it brief: "If I call you to come pick me up, and you're drunk, all you have to say is, 'I can't. I'm drunk.' That's all you have to do. Okay?"

She neither nods nor flops back, and now I know she's drunk. Her driving had me fooled for a while, because she kept it fairly straight until she casually drifted over the yellow line. You hate to grab the wheel at fifty miles an hour, but you can't very well help jolting from your seat and thrusting your hands in that direction with a semi coming at you. She drifts back to our side of the road, casually ignoring me and overly correcting to within an inch of the shoulder. I would tell her to pull over, but she'd resist, and we'd argue, and we have only five miles to go. So I merely take the beer from her cup holder. We make it home, and there's no point in yelling now. Still, I'm upset. Now she can't hide her condition at all, half-staggering and driveling nonsense.

"Esh .... Esh he can't scoll a prasht."

"What?"

"A prasht. He can ... can ... t! ... shcoll a. . . . "

"I can't understand you. You're not making sense. You're not speaking in sentences."

"Ish. Ish him prasht an. . . . "

"What did you have to drink?" She can't remember. She doesn't actually say that she can't remember, but her face slowly twists in the cornered agony of a sauce-head, busted. "Tell me how many drinks you had. I want to know. You had plenty. I know you did. What was it? Did you drink a bottle of wine? Two bottles? Or was it vodka? Don't tell me you got this sloshed on beer." I'm not yelling. I'm admirably calm. I don't want to stick her nose in it, but she should at least see the consequence of drinking and driving.

"I din .... I din.... dring.... "

"Yeah, right. You had a beer open when you picked me up. And here's another one in your hand. That's two. Two beers. What do you call two beers? Lawn furniture? I've seen you soak up four or six and stay clear. So I know you had plenty."

"I din .... I din ... Shum ... shumsing ... wrong wiss me .... I hah .... I hah.... diss pain.... "

"You have a pain?" She nods. "Where? Where is the pain?"

She rubs her temple, left side. "Here. Reay bah. Shafternoo. I randa gate when everybuy one time, an'en shree time. . . ."

"Hey." I set a hand on her headache. She lowers her head as if to let me feel the pain. I don't think something is amiss, but that's because I'm hungry. And it's late, nearly eight o'clock already. "Sh. Go lay down. I'll make dinner. We'll check it out tomorrow."

"Ish wrong. Li'l shings." Her arms rise weakly. Her fingers flutter. "I shee. Buh whe look it. Goh. Shumshing wrong wiss. . . ."

"It's okay. We'll take care of it. Tomorrow morning. Go relax now. I'll make dinner. Okay?"

"Oke. . . . Okay."

"You're telling me you had nothing to drink?" She half nods in response. "Nothing? Not one thing?" She nods again. "Except for two beers." She stares.

Two beers my ass. Then again, this is either the most drunk I've seen her, or it's something else. I've seen her slur but never mince. Well, we'll check it out in the morning, first thing. We can't do anything now, even if something is amiss. But I don't think it is, and even if it is, she's better off here than in a waiting room all night.

Besides, her color is good, temperature normal, and look; already she lies on the sofa fast asleep, oblivious to Larry King Live and my famous barbecued chicken, coming right up. I prep dinner and go to the living room, where I cover her with the knit comfort. I proceed with yellow squash and an excellent salad with mixed greens, feta, olives, some thin-sliced purple onion and vine-ripe tomato, the first of the season. On top will be olive oil, fresh-squeezed lemon juice and crushed garlic. Oh, we do eat well. It accounts for the vitality around here, not to mention our natural immunity.

I think she's drunk. I quickly check the bottom cabinet under the toaster for an easy answer—for a pint of vodka or a half-dead soldier of moderately priced wine. I find none, but I think she's drunk. Anyway, we can't do anything now. She's sleeping soundly. She's warm and looks peaceful. I cover her again with another blanket. What the hell can you do at eight o'clock at night? Hit the emergency room for a nice six-hour chat with the winos, derelicts, crash victims, knife and gunshot wounds? Jesus. Sit in the fluorescence while a teenager behind a cheap desk drills you on the history of disease in your family and the fine-print caveats in your insurance policy? I don't think so. Hell, that can't be the same as quiet repose, and we wouldn't see a doctor until morning anyway, so we'll wait. Dinner will be ready in no time. But I'd bet a dollar to a donut she sleeps through, through the bake and last ten minutes, when I brush the sauce on. I think she might be drunk. It's the only thing that takes her out like this.

I'm right again; she sleeps through. Well, maybe she'll wake up hungry, so I leave dinner on the stove. The barbecued chicken is one of my best.

She wakens near ten. I monitor sobriety, and I'm affirmed, I think. She seems iffy. She doesn't get hung over, ever, but she seems dazed, like after a nap on a hot summer day. "Dinner is excellent," I say. "It's on the stove. Are you hungry?"

"Mm. Yes," she says, rising and going, shuffling things around and coming back but not with dinner. She has only a cup of ice cream.

"That's all you want?"

She smiles. "Mm. Hmm."

"How do you feel?"

"I don't know. I feel okay."

"No headache?"

She shakes her head.

We sit and watch the box. It babbles. I press the mute. "Rachel." She turns. "I need you to tell me something." She waits. "I won't be pissed off. Okay?" She waits. "Tell me exactly what you had to drink."

"When?"

"All day. All night."

"I already told you. Two beers." She hits the volume control to restore the sound and hits the channel selector for 34, *Real TV for Real Women*, her favorite. Well, she only had two beers and that's good, actually, because tomorrow is the seventeenth, St. Pat's, and we've planned an outing to town to help fend off the fidgets of a tardy spring. We've frankly had it with the cold and wet, and a day of the blarney will remedy what ails us, at least in the short run. Then we'll be that much closer to warmer weather.

Tomorrow's outing will be a spiritual exercise as well. Maybe I only justify a daytime drunk of my own; but I have a theory that the lost tribe of Israel may be Irish, and I think insight may be gleaned from a child of Ireland, a bartender perhaps, one with a brogue, who might have an opinion on the facts. To whit: Judah Maccabee and his sons rode for eight days and nights to fetch more oil for the Everlasting Light in the Temple in Jerusalem, because the light must never go out, even if Philistines ransack the place and let the oil burn down to a single day's supply. Today we have the Maccabean Games to commemorate the valor of Judah Maccabee and his sons, who rode eight days for more oil, and when they returned, the light still shone. This amazing ride against all odds reminds us that the light can shine everlasting, no matter what.

Okay, drop an e from Maccabee; you get MacCabe. Okay, McCabe, which may be more Scot than Irish, but Ireland is the richest nation in all of literature and close enough to Wales. And Ireland presents a Jew as its most notable literary character. Does not the spirit of Leopold Bloom reach out to every man and woman who ever tilted a pint? Yes, I think yes, again yes.

Green beer, black beer, cloudy beer; you name it; we'll raise it for the Light Everlasting and the spirit you come to love. I might click my heels. If the wife only had two beers, she'll be all the fresher for a proper tribute to Ireland, home of our long lost cousins after all—mine by blood, hers by marriage.

But worry plagues my sleep like a mosquito in my ear. If she only had two beers, then why?. . . . Never mind. Give peace a chance, John Lennon said. Leave them alone, and they'll come home, wagging their tails behind them, someone else said. Give it a rest, I think.

Sure enough, she wakes up chipper as a meadowlark on a fencepost singing out for sunrise in springtime. Up with no doubt and down to feed the dogs and cats, she's soon up again to announce a most extraordinary day. It's clear and sunny. Put that with prospects for an outing in town and a lovely buzz from the freshest beer in the world, and the day shines bright indeed. "What time shall we go?" she asks.

"I don't know, but soon, I think. We don't want to be late. You know what happens when we get a late start. We're so pressed to catch up."

"Okay. So when? Nine? Ten?"

"Maybe noon. I'm going to call what's-his-name. Maybe they can slip you in. We'll stop on the way."

"What's his name?"

"You know. He's not a doctor but he's like a doctor."

"What for?"

"What did you have to drink yesterday?"

She slows down and looks sad. "I had two beers. And there was something wrong with me. I never get headaches but I had this terrible headache, and everyone was showing up at once, so I had to run out to the gate three times in a row. And I was staining the bookcase, and I think the fumes caused it. That's all. I took two aspirin and it went away."

"You took two aspirin?"

"Yes. And I had these things. You know. I could see things over to the side."

"You mean peripherally?"

"Yeah. That's what I said. But when I looked, they weren't there."

"You've never taken aspirin in your life."

"Yes I have."

"When?"

"I took it once."

"Ah, what the hell. What's-his-name'll take twenty minutes. If he takes any longer we'll leave."

"What can he do?"

"Bang your knee with a rubber mallet and ask you the same questions I asked."

"We don't need to do that."

"I know we don't."

"I'm fine now. I feel fine."

"You look fine. And you sound well."

She often accuses me of subtle manipulation to maintain control like this, agreeing with her but not really listening, as if my thoughts alone are valid. I assure her she taught me everything I know of passive control. But the day is too bright for petty argument, so we move forward with an herb tea for her and a double-tall latté for me, for the feeling.

Bill Varne is a physician's assistant, not a doctor, but he looks like, talks like and acts like a doctor. He bangs her knee and asks what she had to drink. He asks about the headache and the aspirin. He wants to know if she still sees movement over to the side and if neurological disorder runs in her family. She answers cleanly down the line. Strong goyishe stock sounds harsh, but the truth is often blunt. She can be knocked down, but she won't stay down. I've seen her bounce back in hours from the flu. Cuts and bruises heal overnight. Oh, she's a health nut all right. Bill Varne says she's fine. Good, we're on our way. I think I'll skip brunch to better prime the system for an easier buzz and some world-famous corned beef and cabbage. Rachel can get some spring rolls or a salad. Or maybe she'll try the cabbage.

"I'm going to get you in down at Davidson Hospital in Bremerton, near the Naval Shipyard."

"Hospital?"

"For a CAT scan. You really should."

"I feel fine."

"You look fine. So why not?"

"Because. We're going to Seattle. We have it planned."

He shrugs with a wry smile. "Wait here."

When he's gone, she stands up and says this is a waste of time. She feels fine. Let's go. I agree, averse to losing a day of healthful benefits for no purpose other than to generate some billings. Of course we're cynical, but our jaded perception of the medical industry is ingrained from experience; moreover, we crave the day ahead, as planned. We manage to reach agreement on keeping this short and sweet. In no time Bill Varne returns with the good news: nobody gets a CAT scan around here in less than two days, but he got us in at two-thirty.

"Two-thirty?"

"Yes. Isn't that great?" He doesn't exactly smile but conveys that iffy, hopeful look.

"Look. I can do this Friday. Okay?"

Now he smiles, but it's the smile of no smile. I sense a soft close on products and services based on apprehension/anxiety, but I go along with Mr. Varne. "Hey. It's on the way," I say.

"On the way? It's twenty miles south."

"But it isn't till two-thirty. So we have time to get there. And I really do have some calls to make this morning. And we've never ridden the Bremerton Ferry. So big deal. Then we can take our time and relax. Besides, it's fun to hurry and catch up. I think it could be my favorite."

Bill Varne leaves. "You're so controlling," she says. "I feel fine."

"Humor me," I say, stepping away and out the door and down the hall to catch Bill Varne. I ask, "Is this critical?"

"Oh, yes."

"You didn't see anything."

"That's right. But you had a clinically significant event. You must do this."

I think Bill Varne is a good guy, but I bristle at the language of clinical significance, because I don't consider us to be part of the statistical data set, because we eat extremely well and stay severely active, which, in its own right, seems at least removed and likely independent from and perhaps superior to the double-blind standard. I pause on the brink of telling him who we are, what we've done and the belief system we subscribe to. Ah, hell: he doesn't care, and I'd just as soon be sure on this one rather than make another precious point. We've come this far, so we'll go a bit farther. We've never ridden the Bremerton Ferry, and I do have some calls to make. We have the time. And she only had two beers.

3

—◆◆◆—

Will You Get Away From Me?
Just Get the Fuck Away!

We are thirty miles down the road at the CAT scan place across from Davidson Hospital near the Naval Shipyard in Bremerton. I have made my calls and tidied my desk, tying things up for an indefinite distraction, perhaps, or maybe only preparing for an outing in town. It's hard to pinpoint the time at which your life makes the turn from simple pleasure to ghastly surrealism—and it is a hairpin turn with no gentle curvature. We arrived at two-fifteen for our two-thirty appointment. Rachel went back for her CAT scan at three. I am not allowed back there but shouldn't mind, because, well, just look: here is TV to engage, soothe and sedate me.

I'm watching a renowned editor of a magazine for girl readers who want to look like, talk like and be like the exotic women on the pages of this magazine. The magazine has been an impulse item at grocery store checkouts for decades. The editor is old and wealthy, and her opinion is presumed to be worthwhile.

She explains her fundamental adherence to simplicity; she's done nothing more than go the extra mile to compete successfully in a very tough market. She's rouged like a working girl and every facial surgery available has stretched her skin thinly across her skull. Cavernous eye sockets are underscored, lined and highlighted in vampish blue green, and her cheeks glow with a bony haze. She bats her lashes with the old magic. No, it wasn't power or money that drove her. It was simply simplicity, because she was only a simple girl who did her best, and frankly, she still is. She titters. She looks disinterred, dead these last few years but dug up for a heart-to-heart. She grins in ghastly flirtation, proving the Grim Reaper can be a femme fatale. Fabulous hair surrounds the death head like a bouffant in straw and spray lacquer. It's simple and perfect, like her. This is why I avoid reflection on the world and its ways; they lead to such difficult inference.

What must this old woman see in the mirror? Don't her friends advise her on aging gracefully and letting go the foolishness? We take a break for these important messages, in which the actual moment, location, circumstance and my own denial creep in. I should have been drunk and well fed two hours ago. I should be clicking my heels on a happy stagger home for an afternooncap and blessed abandon with my wife, who still loves my attention and admires my stamina. Yet I sit in a waiting room while she is scanned. Twenty minutes later I stroll to the reception desk, where I ask, "Can you tell me how to get to the Bremerton Ferry?"

"Oh," the receptionist says, glancing at another woman who rifles the file cabinet.

"Oh," says the file cabinet woman. "They can give you those directions over there."

"Over where?"

"Just over there." She points out the door. "You're parked in the lot? Okay, go out the exit and go left and up the drive a hundred yards and turn right and park in front."

"What's over there?"

"The hospital. You need to go right over."

I think this is it, the moment of seeing. I feel a seed suddenly crack and reach out with germination, but I press to know what these people have planned for me and mine. Why must we go right over there? I am told that everything will be explained over there, and they exchange another glance. I feel squeezed in the rough interface between my right to know and the American Medical Association's agenda; one is God-given while the other feels unnecessarily embedded in secrecy. I know they don't mean to be secret but only try to avoid legal recourse on wrong information that may well lead to pain and suffering and other sundry chaos. These nurses sense my discomfort. Their glance seems to ask who in their right mind would resist what is best for them. So I ask again, "Can you please tell me why we need to go right over there to the hospital?"

"Just have a seat. Have a seat, please."

"I think I'll stand, thanks." In fact, I think I'll leave this waiting room, because it feels more suitable to relatives who are more willing than I am to surrender the decision-making process. I think I'll proceed to the source to see what's up and get a straightforward answer to a straightforward question. The radiology tech seems service oriented, so I simply ask, "What do you have?"

"I'm only a tech," she says. "Doctor wants to see you. He'll be out in a few minutes. Sit down, please." I don't mean to be so easily irritated, but this dropping of the article feels wrong, intimating that Doctor is like God, and there is only One. She too senses my trouble and shares my fidget.

"Don't you mean *the* doctor?" I ask.

"What?" she asks back.

I want free of this onrush of anxiety and what feels like a house of mirrors. Who wouldn't? Rachel is in the CAT scan room, getting dressed. And just that quickly, I'm out of patience. "Punch it up. Now, please. Chop chop. Let's go."

I step forward with reasonable concern, and she complies, perhaps unsettled by lack of proper authority but willing to go along with a verbal disclaimer. She mumbles, "I'm only a tech," and elaborates on the inconsequential essence of anything she might say. She reminds me that Doctor must say it, if it's to mean anything. The monitor brightens with brain scans as a fellow in his mid-twenties comes out a door down the hall and strides this way. He introduces himself a few paces out, but I can't hear him. The left half of the monitor in front of us is pre-empted by a white mass. I am past the moment of germination in another moment of dramatic growth; the moments divide and grow with sudden acceleration. They pile on with knowing. I am reminded of the old days of lift-off, when I lay back on the sofa gripping the cushions to either side through the G-forces of the LSD experience, so I wouldn't roll off. Just hang on, I told myself. Soon you'll level at altitude. Then you can maneuver, but don't try it just yet, because turns and banks under a load like this can rip your wings off. The little mosquito from last night enlarges like a hallucination. With a growing wingspan and teeth to match, it swoops. This is alternate reality.

I turn to Doctor as he says, ". . . massive cerebral hemorrhage in the left temporal lobe. . . ."

"I feel fine," she says, standing by me now.

"We think this occurred today," Doctor says.

"I'm sure it was yesterday." I don't mean to correct him, because I'm acutely aware of my impression on others.

"Or yesterday," he allows.

"Or maybe a long time ago," I venture.

"No. See the brightness. That means it's fresh."

"You mean the blood?"

He nods.

"When the blood ages, it darkens?"

"Yes. It darkens quickly."

"Like life," I say, at once regretting my outlook and acceptance of the dark spirit. I feel its presence, a tangible solidification in the company we share. Call me superstitious or spiritually aware. I recognize an ethereal population, an air around us jostling with lost and partial souls. Do you think it doesn't exist? I think this place is closed to the world of wonder but dense with forlorn spirits. I think this is a place of double-blind faith; the medical staff apparently senses our discomfort. They stand by to see what we'll do.

Well, we stare at the monitor as if the bartender will surf to another game and we can have another beer. I've known about dark entities for years, which doesn't make me extrasensory; some people are attuned to the ether; some are not. The dark forms avoid delineation, usually by favoring peripheral movement. They disappear when you turn to them straight on, because they're not of this world, not of the flesh. Perhaps they're as queasy as we are in the act of recognition. That's what Rachel saw. Now I sense their proximity. I wonder why and whom and how many. Are they jacked-up and hungry for some innocence? I turn to her. I smile, maybe because she doesn't disappear. "Do you still see them?"

"See what?"

"The peripheral movements."

"Maybe a little bit. But I'm fine. I'm telling you I feel fine. I am fine."

I turn to Doctor, perhaps hoping he'll disappear.

"We need you to go right over to the hospital. Take these with you." He hands us the film negatives. "They're expecting you."

"What will they want to do?"

"I can't say. I can only guess." He hesitates, seemingly aware of his professional dark entity, Liability.

"What would you guess?"

"My guess is that they'll want to medivac Rachel to Seattle. She has a very dangerous condition."

"In a helicopter?"

He nods grimly.

"That's ridiculous. I feel fine. We're going over there anyway. Come on." She grabs the film negatives and is on her way to Seattle. She moves sprightly now on quick, short steps like a woman insulted, or maybe a woman who knows her rights. I hurry to catch up. "What a crock."

"I'll say."

She has a ferry schedule in her purse. "Oh, shit. Now we missed the three-ten."

"Oh, well. We have to drop these off anyway. When's the next one?"

"Not till four-thirty!"

"Plenty of time."

"This is so frustrating. We should be over there right now!"

"We'll go late. What's the rush?"

"Oh. You were looking forward to this."

"Still am," I assure her, lying with unnatural aplomb.

"Let's just go. We'll drop these off on Friday."

I shake my head. "Then I'll have to drive all the way back down. Besides, it's a courtesy." She shakes her head, and before you know it, I've achieved passive manipulation once again as we reach door number three. It opens onto rural bedlam, a hospital emergency room in a military/farm/OK-Used-Cars town.

This is more like it, with a staff more attuned to punctuality, and we don't have to wait at all. In fact, they're expecting us. They whisk us to the inner sanctum, dispensing with the waiting room and its teeming injured yearning to be free. I doubt anyone here has severe cerebral hemorrhage, yet here they sit, when they could be savoring corned beef and cabbage with the best beer in the world. Oh, boy, the choices some people make.

Doctor could have been a fraternity brother of Doctor, I think. He spares us further knee taps and questions, except for having Rachel squeeze his fingers and tell him what month it is, what day of that month and who is President of the United States of America. Rachel squints as if into the mystical realm and tells him March 17th and the year of record and the full given name of the President of the United States of America. He looks puzzled by her apparent sarcasm but lets it pass as he slumps in resignation or bedside manner. Yes, he can sense our view of the process and apprecieate our little joke, but this is not the time for humor. Low and mellifluous he says, "Tell me what happened."

"Well, I was painting this bookcase we have—"

"You mean staining." I only correct her to establish a record.

"Staining. And the door was broken last week and all these people, I think three of them, came to the house right in a row. And I had to drop everything and run out and open the door and then close it—"

"You mean the gate."

"The gate. And then I had to close it so the dogs wouldn't get out. And the smoke from the paint—"

"You mean the fumes. Rachel. He needs to know what happened with your head."

"That's what I'm saying. Let me finish. So the smoke was really, you know, making me all dis.... dis ...."

"Oriented."

"Yes. And I got this splitting headache. And I never take aspirin. So I took two buttons and then I felt easy but I had to go.... And now I see these dots.... These .... See?" She reaches to the side without looking there.

Doctor leans in with gentle certainty. His anxiety underscores my own. As if deferring on cue to the dark spirits whose presence is now official, Rachel has dropped again into wrong words, the first since waking up this morning. The young doctor seems capable enough, except for his visible anxiety over what could be his first drop-dead interview. He grasps her forearm and nods, perhaps hoping we'll nod too. "Have you ever been on a helicopter?" He smiles, maybe hoping we'll share his enthusiasm for the terrific fun ride in our near future.

"Sure," Rachel says. "We used to live in Hawaii. I've been up plenty. I've been over Haleakala—the tornado—and around the backside to Hana. I hate those things."

He smiles. "I want you to take a helicopter ride."

"Why?"

"You've had a massive cerebral hemorrhage. I. ..." He laughs short. "I gotta tell you. Nobody here has ever seen anything like this. Why aren't you in a coma?"

"Why can't you relax?" she asks back. "I feel fine. We're not going for a helicopter ride."

"We don't want *him* to go," Doctor says.

"Don't want me to go?"

"You can take the ferry or drive around. No family or friends can go in the helicopter."

"Oh, you're dreaming." She says it, not me; yet I understand her resistance to the offer. "You think I'm locking up with you guys with no protection?"

"What's the rush?" I ask.

"You're wife is . . . . Well, she's at extreme risk. She could drop dead any second. *A sneeze could kill her!*"

I find myself nodding, not so much with new realization but with a hammering in of the old.

"That's ridiculous. I feel fine. We have maps. It's four o'clock, and we haven't had anything to eat."

"You just. . . . can't. . . ." Doctor is very flustered.

"Please. Doctor, can you give us a couple minutes?"

"All right." He sits there.

"Alone."

"Oh."

He leaves. Rachel babbles that she is not, repeat not, at extreme risk, because she feels fine. If she didn't feel fine, that would be another movie, meaning story, but she suspects the helicopter concession here thrives on customers in coma, who cannot resist. We can take these scratch scan film thingies to wherever they need to go tomorrow. We'll have plenty of time then and a fresh start on a brand new day. In the meantime, she feels fine.

I watch. I listen. And just like that I am holding my face in two hands and sobbing. She steps up and cradles my head, she with the massive cerebral hemorrhage. "Jesus. You're ploving a snit. I'm the one with the headache."

"Look. . . ." I struggle to collect myself. "You're going to have to help me out on this. I know how you feel about what kinds of things go on here. But I can't do this alone."

"Do what alone? We're not doing *anything*."

"I agree. No helicopter. We'll catch the ferry and drop these off at the hospital."

"That's what you said before. We're at the hospital. So why go to another hospital? There's nothing wrong with me."

"Rachel. You've had a massive cerebral hemorrhage. Don't you get it?"

"I feel fine."

"I know you do. And I'm proud of you. But we must go to the next step. You're dropping words. Are you aware of that?"

She hangs her head. "This is so bad." Then she rubs her left temple.

"Yes. And it may get worse. In the meantime, please move slowly and talk softly. I can't. . . . I can't do this alone."

She hugs me again. "Okay. Can we leave now?"

I nod and we exit the inner sanctum. We hail Doctor and tell him our plan. He offers a few short gasps of disbelief and shakes his head and says to wait here. I tell him with cold certainty that we have no time to spare, so we will be on our way in one minute. He nods. He steps back and behind the front desk, then back again. Without moving his left foot, he seems disturbingly similar to Curly Joe. He has a clipboard with consent forms. He wants us to sign off.

"You're confused," I tell him. 'We're not taking the helicopter."

"I know. This just says that you understand your wife is at extreme risk and may die on the way over. She may die on the ferry. She may have a stroke that will leave her without speech. But it might not effect her cognizance, so she'll know she's impaired with no hope of recovery."

"How can you ask us to consent to something we're not doing? You make this feel like a Kafka story. Do you know Kafka? He was a doctor too, and he wrote stories like this one."

"I haven't read him, but I know who you mean. Please, this is my career on the line. I can't let you go without. . . . I mean; you have nothing to lose here. I mean. . . . You know what I mean." He's nearly as unsettled as I am, and he adequately conveys his heartfelt need in troublesome times. We both sense death perched on the rafters ready to pounce. The reassembly of a shattered life would follow for both of us by way of deep, personal loss and the investigation that would surely begin. How could this have happened with rational people on hand?

She died on the ferry? But she was in the Bremerton ER! You let her walk out?

"I do know what you mean. You want to save your ass even though we're not willing to save ours." He offers the tight-lipped smile in difficult agreement. "Let me ask you something else, though. Don't you worry about pressure changes?"

"Pressure changes? She's already bled. The pressure won't change again unless she bleeds again." He jots something down, perhaps noting that I too display symptoms of confusion and speech pathology. Then again, my floating doubt is out of the hole at planing speed, and with momentum comes paranoia. Maybe he only jotted an innocent reminder to get the milk, bread and eggs on the way home.

"Pressure changes at altitude."

He glares at me and suddenly sees. "Oh! Well, no, not really. It doesn't work that way. For one thing, they don't go very high at all."

"Do they go higher than sixty feet? You know it's easy going up, but rough coming down."

He puffs in exasperation. "It doesn't work that way."

"Why not?"

"Because she's not embolized. And you have no air pockets in your head so the pressure is already equal. A hemorrhage doesn't emit air of any kind into the space, and liquid cannot change volume, which is what you're suggesting."

"What about the Eustachian tubes that run up to the inner ear? Can you feel them on descent? And how do you know she's not embolized?" Embolism is the blocking of a blood vessel that causes everything on the pressure side of the block to swell. It results from aberrant flow or off-gassing with no decompression following a deep dive, which is another example of dramatic pressure change. Embolism occurs in a weak system or a combination of the above conditions. Eustachian tubes do conduct air and constrict under pressure, which you feel on descent of any flight. You get relief from dilation, which can be effected with a nose blow or a sneeze or a yawn, none of which seem sympathetic to a cerebral hemorrhage. Certified divers and snorkel executives are sensitive to ambient pressure, below the surface or above.

Doctor wants to present his side of the story but hardly has time because we just don't get it, and we may have a death here momentarily, and he's very busy with people who want his help, so please.... He slides the consent form and pen toward me, and I sign. Because we all need to move along. This isn't the first or last thing he or I wouldn't agree on. It doesn't matter. He half nods and offers the pen to Rachel. She signs as well and says it's time to go. He wishes us luck, like a cashier at Vegas, and he's off to the more receptive.

We're out the door, in the car and on our way, but we're not exactly sure how to get there. The dogs whine. Molly has to pee. Oh, yeah, we have Molly and Dino with us, because they can't spend the night alone, because Molly has to pee. And if we have too much fun and can't manage the long trek home, we can camp in town at my office on the ninth floor. I'm a distributor of masks, fins and snorkels, who would much rather be researching a distant reef with my assistant. But the clouds roll in.

I turn the key and the dashboard bongs and flashes, signaling *Time for Service!* I press a few buttons to make it stop but to no avail. I want to kick the dashboard but can't get my foot in place, but in a minute it stops. Rachel tells the dogs to hold it; we have to make the ferry. She explains to them that we'll most likely have a few minutes wait in the holding area, and then we can all take a leak. Molly licks her excitedly.

But I can't find the Bremerton Ferry, and it takes an hour and twenty minutes to cross anyway. So we scratch that plan for a ride up to Bainbridge, which takes thirty minutes to drive, but then that ferry is only forty-five minutes in crossing Puget Sound, and besides, we can stop at Central Market on the way for some sushi—her idea. She seems out of touch, rising in my esteem in the face of extreme risk. She's hungry. She wants sushi. She will eat. What a woman.

I beg her to wait in the car, but no. She'll let the dogs pee then shag the beer while I get in line with the sushi. "Beer? You want beer?"

"I will. And you want some. Don't you?"

"Yes. Get six."

We make the ferry on time. On board we eat and agree; the sushi is very good. I inhale a beer and crave another but by now the dark spirit crowds me, reaching in and tying knots in my gut and head at will. I sense another difficult interface, this one between my health-nut wife on the one hand, and the American Medical Association up ahead on the other. She only yesterday took the first two aspirin of her adult life. She eats no red meat and hardly any fish or chicken. She knows an antioxidant from a free radical and understands the beneficent nature of bioflavonoids and the innate danger of polyunsaturated fat.

She believes we are now engaged in a nuisance, that we'll soon be on our way, sloshing green beer, black beer, many beers, having a grand Irish time in town. She pulls a new compact disk from my glove box, a digital re-recording of Billie Holiday's greatest hits. "I got you this," she says. "If anything happens to me, and you don't like it, take it back to Fred Meyer's. The receipt's in there." I scan her for sincerity but need not look too deep. She hates wasting money. At least she recognizes the potential here, even if casually, in passing humor. Then again, I really can't tell if that's her strength showing or her lunacy.

I'm amazed at this juncture how the milestones arise and connect, in this case her subtle reference to a refund on a Billie Holiday CD and the realization that we're heading casually over to Seattle for brain surgery. We don't want surgery of any kind and in fact have a history of declining surgery, yet surgery will be served up with no option. This knowing comes on like gangbusters—on the certainty of brain surgery with no option I would bet the farm. Yet I repress. I side with my wife. Do we not know what we have learned? Is there not another way, what the American medical complex so deftly calls an alternative? Is not every invasive procedure balanced by another, more sane approach? I think so. Yet I fear the entities whipping my periphery, emboldened by such a grip. Of course what I feel is fear. It holds form when I turn to look: Puget Sound is gunmetal gray and frothy white with gusts to fifty knots. Spindrift swirls and smacks the windshield.

"Better get the car mushed," she says. She means washed but winces sweetly in compensation for her mistake.

"Look," I say. "I need to call Sue." Sue is her sister who expresses herself freely and stays extremely busy with her children and family concerns. Sue is plugged into two-twenty and makes Rachel appear to be complacent.

"No! Are you kidding? You're making this into some kind of big deal, and I'm telling you it's not!"

"Listen." She's listening. I'm not sure how to tell her the truth that is now so evident, that they will want her to check in, and I may agree with them, but I will never go along with brain surgery, not now or ever, without her consent. No, don't even mention surgery. "I'm going to need help on this."

"Help? With what?"

"They may want you to stay the night."

"Do you know what happens in there?"

"I'll stay with you. I won't leave you alone. But I have to drop the dogs off. We can't leave them in the car. I have to call Sue so she can stay with you while I drop the dogs. Please. Please go along with me on this."

"I don't like it. I don't like it one bit, and you're making it worse."

"I don't want to make it worse. I don't know what else to do. I need your faith. You must believe that I can get you out of this as soon as possible. Please."

She mumbles; out of what? What is it that anyone needs out of? I dial Sue. I keep it brief, but the operative phrase sets Sue off. "Cerebral hemorrhage! Do you know what that is? . . . . " Yes, yes, yes Sue; we know what that is. Sue will be down as soon as she can.

Finding a parking place feels miraculous, as if events are random and extreme with a will of their own; who could ever anticipate a cerebral hemorrhage or a parking place in downtown Seattle? We walk Molly and Dino down the block for another pee. Rachel thinks this unnecessary; they only just peed an hour ago, and we'll be done here in what? Twenty, thirty minutes?

What the hell, I explain; sometimes I have to pee every hour. And besides, we don't want to be rushed. We want to do this right so we won't be bothered again, so we can get on with our St. Pat's, our beer, our fun and our lives. I'm speaking to her like a parent to a child. To my chagrin, she accepts my explanation.

We give Molly and Dino water in their dish. And when Molly walks a short distance and squats for a massive dump, a surly fellow much bigger than me walks by and says, "Where's your fucking plastic bag."

I surprise myself with dynamic range, displaying street diplomacy off the cuff, at night. "If I had one it would go over your head," I tell him with practiced certainty, because ambient pressure has built up subtly and now seeks the smallest opening through which to ventilate. This is only one more hazard of changing pressure. I regret my behavior, not for reasons of etiquette or personal development but because a brawl could significantly inconvenience us just now. But the surly fellow perceives our need to move along and leave a few dog turds in the grass, which, after all, will go away much quicker than all these cars or even a single plastic bag.

He mumbles something about assholes and dog shit on public streets and keeps walking. I agree with him on all levels. We tuck the dogs back in and explain to them, "Stay. You stay. Stay."

And hand in hand under a clear, starry night in Seattle in early spring we stroll down the promenade. She smiles my way. "Don't get all fluster-caked in here. Okay?"

"Fluster-caked?" She gives me the look that says to bug off. "I'll try my best," I say. "You can help, you know."

"They just better not try to mess with me."

"Damn straight," I agree. What a woman. We approach the marquis, *Emergency Room*, and the big double doors. Several people of the street are outside in hospital-issue pajamas. Each stands beside a portable intravenous feedbag rack on wheels, with a monitor and injection tubes in their forearms. One smokes a cigar. Two are lighting butts, hardly used. One scratches her butt. They all need a shave. "Well, here we are again," I say. Rachel looks up. "Walking through life together."

"Pshh."

A squat young woman with sallow skin sits inside behind a window with a talk hole. She asks our name and address and insurance program and employer and on and on down her list to, "Are you an organ donor?"

"That's premature. Can we let you know?"

"I have to fill this in," pleads the receptionist.

"No," I tell her.

"Yes. I am." Rachel smiles. She's not attached to the flesh and likes the idea of giving to make a difference.

I remind her, "You know they get excited in here. They'll take your spleen if you don't belch on time."

She shrugs. "I just want to get this over with."

Me too. So we answer mechanically to questions of name, age, address, diseases in the family, insurance carrier and type of coverage and who will guaranty payment if the insurance company reneges. With documentation clearance we are signed off on accuracy, truth in lending and indemnification of all debt herewith and forevermore, and so we enter what feels like the Valley of the Shadow—what feels like the wrong place for us, the uniquely healthy.

Six rows of gurneys stretching to the horizon can make you smile and think that there must be some mistake here, that we are not part of this. A hundred people in blue scrubs scrabble among the drunks, droolers, crashes, burns, heart attacks, assaults, batteries, knife fights, gangbangs and the generally mortally forlorn. We have entered the single Trauma Center servicing the five nearest states. States of the union, that is; states of consciousness are wider ranging, favoring the shrill end of the spectrum. Wailing is universal and rises like a chorus. Moaning is the refrain. The staff is a study in movement, fast but slow, orderly, chaotic, non-stop, driven, dedicated, caffeinated, compulsive and gratified.

The blue team doesn't drop a beat but injects, cuts, squeezes, slices, pokes, wraps, swabs and otherwise strives to contain the world of squirming flesh around us. Pulse is everything, and it also rises in waves from the blur of activity. Human industry and agony meet in cross currents; the wave breaks forever in a din of white noise so profuse you must yell to be heard. Or maybe it's just the excitement that raises our voices. The best beer in the world and corned beef and cabbage are only down the hill and around the corner but a world away. This is not what is seen on TV. This is as different from showbiz as three dimensions are different from two. Or four. This has teeth that rip and tear at composure for the newly arrived. All join in the frantic sense of urgency, as if it's contagious and airborne.

A nurse strides forward. She is bigger than me, possibly three of Rachel, and she comes on, as strong as the giant just down from the beanstalk, busy, late and peeved. She grabs the film negatives, pulls them out, nods once, states a wrong name and says, "Finally. You made it. We didn't think you would."

"That's not us."

She holds up the negative. "This isn't you?"

"That's us. You said, 'Jones.' We're not Jones."

"Psh. Never mind. Come over here, Sweetie."

"Where?"

"Right here."

The big nurse wears a nametag: BETTY. Betty is big but not fat, and she wears her hair in a butch. "Squeeze my fingers. Okay. What month is this? Who's the President?"

"You mean the President of the United States of America?" Rachel toys with authority, and I think it a good sign that she's holding her own. Betty glares and hunches low. I read the blitz and tell Rachel to squelch the levity. *Oh, baby,* Betty's body language seems to say; you wanna tango? Well, come on then.

Betty wears three ball bearings in one ear and one in the other. Moving smoothly as a time-lapse sundown, she smothers Rachel with a hug, reaching behind for shirttails and a sweater hem. She is undressing my date, who tells her, "Stop it. What are you doing?"

"Tell me what happened," Betty says, unfastening Rachel's pants and dropping the zipper. "Slip out of these." Betty works it like a puppeteer, deft at disrobing a patient. Rachel goes along with hopeless resistance, babbling about the bookcase, the fumes and the sheep, meaning dogs, the many people arriving at the house, one after the other, and the aerobic push to meet their needs down the hall, meaning the driveway, at the gate. She sees things out there to the side and points to them as she is quickly wrapped in a green seersucker gown too big for Betty.

"Okay, here," Betty says, leading the patient to the gurney and firmly guiding her onto it. "Lay yourself down right here."

Rachel stops, a certain rock in a rising stream, and she explains to Betty, "We're not staying here."

Betty meets this resistance with a sudden grin of lumberjack proportion while easing her own body briefly from tension to camaraderie. She takes a rare breath uncluttered with words and says, "Of course you're not. I just need you to help me out with this for a few minutes. Then we'll get you out of here as quick as we can. Okay?"

Those are my lines. But I sense alliance with Betty. She sees these symptoms as often as not—the denial and resistance. Though I doubt she often sees such a patient who knows a thing or two. And though I like big Betty, she feels too hurried on a fixed agenda designed to serve a group called average that, in our world, generates stats factoring into a woefully low denominator. That is, we should not be likewise factored, because, because.

I strive for etiquette if not good taste, to hide my distrust. I am on—on guard, on alert, on the ready to stand forward and stop the juggernaut. I have heard what they can do. I am doubtful that a machine like this with so many cogs can cohere at this level without a misfire. Well, of course it can't, and that's the basis of our apprehension—that and medical malpractice, medical jurisprudence and medical associations, beginning with the American, with its codes, practices, policies and safeguards.

I will not lose sight of our faith in the human body to heal itself. Call it the God within or homeostasis. We understand what a very small percentage of the viewing audience at home understands, because we've taken the time to learn these things. Betty doesn't know that about us, but she'll learn, as soon as we can chat. It shouldn't take long, say a minute or two.

You might think a woman so liberated, as Betty appears to be, would understand that some people are different. Don't many women agree that only a woman can properly know what a woman feels? I thought they did. Yet Betty leads the next charge, interrupting Rachel in mid-sentence as Rachel explains the need for a door at the end of the hall so the sheep won't get out, you know, in the thing. Betty dives in with two intravenous spikes to the right forearm and a hearty accolade, "My God! You have gorgeous veins!"

Rachel sits up to protest but Betty pins her back with one big paw in the center of the chest. "Lay back, Sweetie. I need these to keep your pressure up." Betty's behavior seems forward if not obtrusive. We haven't even begun our chat.

Rachel whimpers, but not from pain. Her pain threshold is extraordinary. More than tolerance to pain is her good cheer in the face of blood and gore.

In a few short hours she'll have her scalp parted with a nine-inch incision so it can be peeled back to expose a three-inch section of her skull. That section of skull will be removed with a remarkable little buzz saw so the left temporal lobe of her brain can be lifted by hand, so the clot can be removed, and a titanium clip will be fastened to the blood vessel with the aneurysm. She will listen to the plan. She will ask why she needs general anesthesia just for that. The "team" will laugh at her question, but she'll wait for an answer. When she gets none, she will rail, and they will note once again her paranoia. But I get ahead of myself.

Betty rounds the gurney in two strides, grabs the other arm and wraps it tight in a blood pressure bladder. The bladder inflates. Betty explains that we shouldn't worry, because this pressure monitor is automatic and will inflate every few minutes. Meanwhile, she grabs the left wrist with a vice-like grip and pokes first the wrist and then the forearm with two more spikes on plastic tubing.

Rachel is a munchkin next to Betty but rises to the occasion by throwing the big nurse off. I am neither proud nor embarrassed but rather stunned. Engaging in fight-or-flight response and fortified with adrenaline, Rachel achieves the strength of an opposing linebacker. This is natural, and she's no weakling in the first place. What stills our frantic little radius and tinges the air with dark laughter is her sudden metamorphosis. No word-dropping here, she speaks with clarity, with volume and strength that resonates round the arena. "Will you get away from me?" Heads turn: for the first time, she is heard. "Just get the fuck away!" She is trembling now and changing color.

Big Betty moves in, moves back, goes side to side and calls me away. Maybe now, I think, we can get to know each other and make an informed decision after viewing the unique needs of the individual patient and the options at hand. Is that not reasonable? How much time could it take?

4

Doogie Howser

Betty is up to the action. Hardly discouraged, she leads me to the periphery of our space five feet away. This short distance insulates us from eavesdropping by the difficult patient. Betty says I must now take over.

"Take over what?"

"She's demented. She's irrational. You're going to have to make some decisions here."

"It sounds like the decisions were made before we got here. Betty, we need to talk to somebody. We don't mind talking to you. Or we can talk to a doctor. We need information, plain and simple. We're perfectly willing and able to make decisions, but we don't know what our choices are. Nobody has told us. Can you tell us?"

Betty shakes her head, marginally hiding her impatience. In two strides she's back with the difficult patient. She simply touches Rachel's cheek gently and says, "Sweetie, if we have to give you anything quick, you'll be glad these are in place. We can pump anything we want into your system now in less than three seconds flat."

"We're leaving!" Rachel says. "Take these things off me!"

"Listen. We're going to get you out of here as soon as we can. Just be quiet for a little while." Betty glances around as if checking the perimeter. "Then we're going upstairs for an infusion CAT scan. That'll tell us exactly what's going on."

"What's an infusion CAT scan?" I ask.

Betty takes another step back and another to the side. Three feet instead of five now insulate us, but she's tired of pussyfooting around, and the agony audio is up. "It's just like the first CAT scan, but this machine is more sophisticated. It gives us much more information. Besides, we'll inject her brain with iodine for more detail."

"They said we'd get an MRI. We don't want an infusion CAT scan. We don't want anything invasive. We want an MRI." MRI is magnetic resonant imaging. It's different than a CAT scan because it shows more detail, but not as much detail as an infusion CAT scan with an iodine injection, I think. Betty explains the difference between MRI and infusion CAT scan and the detail provided by each. I tell her we're very comfortable with less detail if it means avoiding the iodine infusion to the brain, and I ask when, in this process, do the patients and families gain the benefit of discussing the options.

She smiles and walks away toward three new crash victims. "That's not my decision to make," she says. "Doctor is on his way."

"Yes, well, we'd like to know a few things." But Betty is out of range, tending to the more receptive. I stoop to Rachel who is now acutely upset. "He's on his way," I tell her. "They want to do an infusion CAT scan. I'll see if we can't substitute the MRI."

"What's an infusion scratch can?"

"It's different. They use a needle."

"I don't want that. I want out of here."

"Patience dear. I'm going full speed."

I set my hand on her arm, high up on the shrinking, unpunctured space remaining. And so we wait with our thoughts and assessments in this world of dramatic reaction. I know they'll press for surgery immediately. It's what they do. And though I know that Rachel is also aware of their drive, she seems still somehow secure in her belief that we're leaving.

The emergency room is big, because this hospital is the single major trauma center serving five states. It feels like an arena, with the roar of a crowd in pain, and athletes of heroic medicine striving to do their best. We feel like the ball. But of course we're traumatized at this point. At any rate, we feel puffy and abused. Rachel's arms are swollen and bruised, and we sense a goal line we're being pushed toward, inexorably stuck in a struggle that is not ours but is between the blue team and the phantom death. Worse yet, the blue team appears to be well seasoned with a game attitude. They hardly fluctuate in pace and emotion in the closing minutes, all tied up against stiff competition. They seem to know and accept that they'll win a few, lose a few; it's the season that counts.

In other times, other terms, this profile might be different, might reflect a dedicated staff attempting to maintain a high standard of survival under difficult conditions and often long-odds situations. The problem at the moment, however, is that analogy is deficient at best; it's not an arena, and the staff are not athletes. We are in a downward spiral, a matrix of apprehension and non-communication; preconceived notions are assumed to be an acceptable substitute for informed dialogue. With no dialogue, no explanation, no options offered, our anxiety is compounded.

Perhaps we're naïve and ungrateful. Or maybe it's the legal system and those pesky consequences of what, in fact, Your Honor, was represented. Of course we are ungrateful, caught between two systems in apparent opposition. I recognize this situation but have yet to engage in any communication, so that I might be corrected or clarified. What will happen next? Who knows? Ultimate faith here is presumed.

Agony is ambient. Wails and shrieks perforate our faint recollection of sanity. Nothing can surprise us. Still, I wonder why such a system so sensitive to legal defense would allow a random orderly to approach us out of nowhere and introduce himself as Michael. I think he must be a part-timer, possibly on a drug-rehab program or otherwise enrolled as a halfway house trusty—or maybe he's working out a community service sentence. I wish him well; he seems civil and lacks only proper diet and exercise to begin his difficult struggle back, to be counted among the living. He appears to be anorexic in his painfully thin and slumped posture, his yellowing and blemished skin suggesting liver malfunction, late acne and mineral deficiency.

He offers his hand, and taking it I am taken with another apprehension. I look up, into his eyes to ascertain that he is not of the phantom entourage. I can't feel it, the hand; like squid under water, it is one with the air around it. I have released flounder with more life than Michael's handshake. He feels intangible, so I release him with care. He says, "Tell me about yourselves." The formally printed name on his tag is defaced by a busy scribble and under that is written: *Michael*. And I realize in another searing moment of knowing, that this is Doctor, another young fellow who only a few summers ago was a sickly kid who wanted to be a brain surgeon.

I want to accept Michael. I want to see him as an eccentrically shaped young man of uncanny skill, but I can't. Of course I'm critical, perhaps acutely so. But I must take responsibility for what happens here, and I can find no confidence. Call me subjective. I'm comfortable with that. I see life as a series of choices that will be based on information and intuition.

Michael displays humility on his chest, what there is of it. He's the same size as Rachel, about a hundred pounds, but he transcends fragility and appears to be eminently, fearfully frail. His voice is a timid lilt like that of Michael Jackson. He's too soft to be heard unless you lean in. I lean in and hear him speak with gentle authority like a man who has found the only calling available to him. His basic social skills seem withered, because he doesn't need the voice or the posture or the appearance of health to answer his calling. He lives in his mind, because he's a brain surgeon. He asks, "Are you new to the area?"

His wary eyes shift in and out of focus, first finding me then looking through me for meaning, real meaning. Are we new to the area? I think he means the Seattle area or one of the five nearby states, though I stumble on another possibility, that he may be referring to the area of rational behavior; are we new to it? Well, clutch situations call for face value, so I tell him we've been in the Seattle area for a few years. Prior to that we were in the Hawaii area for decades. "Ah," he says, nodding sanguinely at the mention of Hawaii. I wonder if Hawaii is known for resistance to what is best. I sense that the word is out on the upscale white couple with a cerebral hemorrhage making trouble on the line.

I see that young Dr. Michael speaks with a heavy lower lip; it drags across his B's and D's and most other consonants like it's filled with sand. I think his embouchure is surgically altered or otherwise short-circuited, perhaps from an aneurysm and cerebral hemorrhage. "Have you been?" I ask. He looks startled. "To Hawaii."

"You know. Everyone is going to Hawaii. Everyone but me. I have no time. I haven't been. But I should go some day."

"If you do, you should be careful. You've had no exposure to the sun." Though Michael's complexion matches the drop ceiling, tepid beige with pockmarks and stains, he reddens, not with a healthy blush but in splotches on his face, neck and chest.

He smiles with practiced patience and murmurs, "I know." I'd like to chat more on fundamental health habits, but we must move on. "Yes. Well. I'm going to examine you. Okay?" Rachel nods, so he plugs his stethoscope into his ears. He wants his fingers squeezed. He wants to know the day and date and current President of the United States. He asks her to hold her arms out, now up, now turn your palms inward. "I'm going to give you three words. Ball. Cake. Metamorphosis. Remember those words. Okay?" He listens there and there and there. "Tell me what happened," he says.

By this time I see the ruse; a talking patient is not a resistant patient. But Rachel is more cooperative and less cynical than I am, so she is spared the difficult view. "I was painting the library. I mean staining. I was staining it. And the . . . the . . . fumes!. . . ."

He taps there and asks for a deep breath. And there. And there. "Do you have any history of cancer in your family?"

"Yes. I was diagnosed with breast cancer."

He stops, opens his eyes wide and asks, "When?"

"Six years ago."

"You had mastectomy?"

"No."

"Radiation?"

"No."

He looks peeved, as if we don't have all day here and nobody is well served by a frickin' guessing game. "What mode of treatment did you choose?"

"And not chemotherapy. There are other ways."

He smiles; he understands. "Hmm. Yes, I'm sure you know about those."

"And I'm sure you don't."

"I'd like to give you a breast exam. Okay?"

"Fine."

But he says, "I'll be right back." He walks away but stops and turns. "Do you remember the three words?"

"I'm. Leaving. Here."

"No. The three words I told you. You don't remember?"

"Ball. Cake. Metamorphosis. Hurry up."

He leaves. Rachel reminds me that we are leaving. She feels fine and wants away right now. Michael is back with another woman from the blue team whose stethoscope dangles from her neck. "Okay. I'm going to give you a breast exam," he says.

Rachel shrugs and nods; he already said that.

"Okay." He looks at the other woman, who nods. Then he slips the green seersucker from Rachel's shoulder to reveal a breast. Two orderlies crane on the periphery. I don't care. Rachel doesn't care. I honestly believe Michael doesn't care. He cops a few feels and covers her back up. The other woman leaves.

"What was that?" I ask. "A political thing?"

Michael reddens unevenly again. I suspect a colleague gave too many breast exams, but I make no comment about a heavy-handed tit man who ruined it for everyone. "No. It's a courtesy. It assures everyone that a breast exam remains a breast exam."

"You guys. . . ." I say, shaking my head.

He rolls his eyes in mutual incredulity and takes notes and then explains the urgent need for an infusion CAT scan. I tell him we don't want a CAT scan. We want the MRI. He says that it's not time for the MRI. I ask why not. He says we need to know the full measure of the aneurysm, whether it's a single or a multiple, whether it burst or simply leaked, where it is and the soundness of the vessels surrounding it. I ask, "The MRI won't tell us this?"

He rolls his eyes again. I sense his avoidance of the answer we both anticipate, which is yes, it will tell us this, which may lead to other questions of a delicate, perhaps legal nature. He says, "Different tests reveal different data. Please, let us do our job. We may need an MRI. And we may opt for an angiogram. Angiogram is the gold standard of detailed information."

"And what is an angiogram?"

"We go in through the femoral vessel in the groin area. We go up through the torso, along the neck and into the brain with optic fiber. It's the only way we can really tell what's going on."

"And that's it?"

"We need two; one clear and one with radioactive dye. It's the second that gives us the gold standard."

"Then why waste time with iodine and no dye? Why not minimize the invasiveness?

"I can explain all these things, but not now."

"If not now, when?"

"Soon. I can tell you this aneurysm popped out yesterday—"

"You mean the hemorrhage occurred yesterday."

"No, I mean the aneurysm occurred yesterday. More can occur today. She's coherent but suffers speech loss. She's not making sense, and we need to do our job."

"I'm sorry, but I disagree with you. She's dropping words, but she's making as much sense as she ever does. She's high energy. She hits the ground running every morning at sunrise. She feeds the animals, works the garden, cooks and cleans. She runs the feral cat program on Bainbridge. In the last year alone she saved a hundred twelve cats."

He rolls his eyes: yeah, yeah, yeah.

"She passes out every night in front of the TV. I watch the rest of the movie, and at bedtime I wake her to go upstairs. Every night she says something like, 'But we can't paint it green. It all goes downhill. And how can we get the garage down from upstairs.' Or something like that. She's done this for years."

"She has?"

"Yes. She has. I think the aneurysm has been there for years. I think it was possibly present at birth."

"How many?"

"How many years has she done this? I don't know. Five or six that I know of."

"Hmm."

"Michael. I think the aneurysm is old. I think it's possibly congenital."

"Hmm."

He ponders, back-pedaling in the inner sanctum, his mind. Of course this is a university hospital, a learning facility that accommodates young students in that amazing transition from adolescence to doctor. So it should be no wonder that I worry over Michael's confidence; he feels dismissive of what I've experienced and know and am willing to discuss. I proceed to explain that we're not part of a statistical average— boy, what a pain in the ass. But we're having a very hard time of accepting this inflexible application of medical school theory with no questions, no dialogue and no inclusion in the process. We understand that we need help, but we think we have choices. We wish he were better versed in alternatives to the scalpel. It's okay with us if he's not up on those alternatives, as long as we can share some rational discourse with mutual respect, which we deem necessary at this juncture.

But Rachel sighs and closes her eyes. I think she can hear me, so I let my insistence go. After all, I'm here to advocate her beliefs and decisions; if she doesn't mind the infusion CAT scan, I should let it be, I think. Everyone feels adversity in the air, but confrontation is not our objective. We in fact regret that we feel necessitated to behave defensively and would like to get on with a more productive exchange. We want to be informed and included, and in fact we require as much, because we won't step blindly into this good night.

I'm confused as well as defensive and must sort my alliances carefully. I can't believe this unusually small, sickly man, yet I can't ignore him.

Adversity feels risky, too close to sudden death. Michael sees his opening, nods, takes a few more notes and says, "We'll be going right up."

Rachel opens her eyes. "What comes after?"

"Angiogram," he says.

"And then?"

"We need to fix you," he says.

"How?"

"It's a simple procedure. We need to remove the clot and clip the aneurysm."

"You mean brain surgery?"

"Well. . . . Yes. That's the only way we can. . . ."

"I'm not having surgery. You can forget that. It's not going to happen."

"Listen. If you. . . ."

"You'll want to shave my head."

"That's right. But you could die any instant. I'm not saying you won't die anyway—"

"We all die someday."

"That's right. You might not die until tomorrow or next week. But I can tell you this: a third of the people with a subarachnoid bleed of this size die instantly. Another third die within the week . . . ."

"You mean here in the hospital?"

"Yes. You may die in surgery. You may have a stroke. You may be severely debilitated any minute. If you don't have surgery, you have a fifty-percent chance of surviving six weeks. Beyond that, you run a five-percent risk of death annually. You're . . . let's see . . . forty-seven. So if you live another twenty years, your risk goes to a hundred percent. It can happen when you're driving down the road or working in the garden. It can happen anytime."

"Hey. It can happen anytime, anyway. And you need to listen to me. I don't believe you. I don't believe anything you say to me. I don't believe you. Do you hear? And you're not shaving my head."

He laughs short. "We won't shave all of it."

"Who'll do the surgery?" She closes her eyes, instantly gaining our attention with a deep sigh. We scan for failure, Michael and I.

She breathes easily, so we proceed. Only moments ago she refused to buy the car, yet now she asks what are her color choices.

Bedside demeanor restored, young Michael assures her, "I will be your doctor."

Rachel opens again and looks at me. I return her gaze, no words necessary. We're old enough to remember the TV series about the regular teenage boy who had to process the rigors of the teen years while—the crux of the drama—exercising his genius for medical practice, which played out each week in a TV hospital, where Doogie Howser was a head surgeon at fifteen, or some such nonsense.

We have no doubt that our very own "Doogie Howser" continues to get excellent grades in school. His complexion may improve, and he may one day have an interest in girls. But he appears to be, in a word, unhealthy. We know the difference between healers and mechanics, and we have a history of choosing the former. This format of urgency and heroic cutting is *why* we have a history of choosing the former—physician, heal thyself and all that. Prospects for a scalpel between Doogie and us are untenable.

"Listen," he says. "You could die any minute. I can assure you. . . ." But he stops short when a nurse steps forward with a new IV bottle. He goes mum as a mob man wary of a wire, as if this nurse is a potential witness. Assurance has been sparse since way back in Bremerton, and I observe that it's doled out in very small dosage and only by those of nurse status or lower.

This pattern will continue to weave. We first sense it casually, then irritatingly. Positive expression must be restrained by anyone above nurse status. Anything beyond a marginal nod can be construed later, in court, as a promise if not a guarantee. Only nurses can dispense compassion and hopeful dialogue, because you can't sue a nurse. Well, you can, but your odds on collected damages are clinically insignificant.

Practitioners may argue that by conveying nothing or a worst-case scenario, they guard against assurance, hope, promise or positive indication in front of witnesses. Positive comments can turn on you in court.

Anything is deniable without a witness. The nurse might be willing to corroborate, and who can take such a chance?

Perhaps this well-intentioned young doctor only safeguards himself and his professional future. That too seems familiar. In serving us he has reminded us many times of potential death but has yet to suggest recovery at any level. "You listen," I tell him. "Please accept what comes your way."

"What?"

"Please. I'm suggesting that you open your mind to a new idea. I think you understand the basis of our hesitation. You seem to be familiar with it at any rate. We'll agree to the infusion CAT scan. Please facilitate that now and leave the rest until later. Let's take this one step at a time. Okay?"

"One step at a time," he back-quotes with a hard stare in classic profile; he will go along with so-called understanding but only with continuing amazement at those who don't know what's best for them. I meet his stare, and soon he nods. Then he fades, drifting ever so gradually backwards. I've seen fish do the same thing, into the murk, for protection.

We will neither see nor hear of him again, ever.

5

An Exercise in Faith

We wait. We recall our experience and faith. Healing is a matter of empowerment; body follows mind. Empowerment comes from confidence, and confidence stems from faith in the face of extreme adversity.

Yes, this is the basis of the fundamentalist Christians who engaged in faith healing not so long ago. That's not to say it didn't work, or, like so many things demonstrating profitability, that it didn't suffer from waves of Charlatan imposters. The fact remains that faith, most notably called the placebo by most doctors, is a known healing agent of formidable power.

But core belief takes a beating in the din and agony, alongside the life and death urgency so constant that it becomes casual. Many big needles perforate that which you hold dear, which is your self, which seems tentatively connected to the world by the little aquarium tubes leading to the electronic brain, flashing and pinging in neurotic fibrillation that seems eerily choreographed with the rest of the sensory onslaught.

Rachel is gripped on the arm at three-minute intervals by the blood-pressure monitor. She is surrounded by an emotionally repressed juggernaut that knows what's best; under siege by superiors, she is told to sit and be still. Rachel says she can't do anything before going to the bathroom. Betty appears from the melee with a bedpan. Rachel tells her to go away and stay away. We wait a few minutes or many, because time is endless; it won't stop and fails to proceed. All that is past is but a moment, like life at the end, seen through a fish-eye lens.

A tall, thin orderly of apparent inner-city descent comes to fetch us up to the infusion CAT scan chamber. His nametag says: *Anthony*. He's different from the others, more relaxed, free of urgency and the need for self-defense. His speech pattern is also uniquely removed from the language of fatal imminence or the probability greater than zero that Rachel will croak at any instant. He alone is attuned to the voice of the mutable object. "I have to pee," Rachel tells him.

"That's easy enough," Anthony says, and we stop down the hall at the bathroom. Her leads are connected to hanging bags and a portable monitor, like a hat rack on wheels. He opens the door and wheels it in then helps her off the gurney and into the bathroom. He is the first to recognize personal dignity and the spoken needs of the patient since our arrival. His demeanor calms us, and a two-minute piss relieves certain pressure. I think he could be fired for his behavior.

In a few minutes we enter the high-tech chamber of the infusion CAT scan. Marginally composed with bladder relief and some respect, we proceed under blazing lights, probing probes and busy hands. The iodine injection goes into her neck. I'm told to leave. I decline. Well, then, wait back there with the technician. But don't say anything. "What would I say?" I ask. But they won't respond to a nuisance.

Wired and primed with Day-Glo, Rachel is fed slowly into the machine. Slice by slice she appears on the monitor till she calls out, "I'm cold! I'm freezing!"

A technician calls back, "Don't move, honey! Don't move now!" The process is halted while Anthony and a woman step out to cover her with a blanket. Meanwhile, the technician at the monitor explains that the iodine is kept cold, so it chills the patient, running up the veins into the brain. I can only imagine; the place is airless as a bunker, causing hot flashes— in me; the staff is apparently adapted. I ponder cold iodine in my veins.

Anthony comes back to the safe area. "Now you get to see what's on her mind," he says.

Her mind is mostly symmetrical except for the low-pressure front building from the east-southeast threatening landfall by midnight. Nurse Betty materializes at my side, in my ear. Gently, she whispers, "You have to take over. She's demented. She has memory loss and depressed speech centers. She's irrational. You need to make the decisions."

I turn and speak clearly, for I, too, may soon call on witnesses in a process that may well judge behavior here. "I will not make a decision for surgery without her approval. I assure you her behavior is no less rational than the scene surrounding us. She is in full possession of her faculties." I wince inside at my own hopeful longing. "I will assist and facilitate where I can. In the meantime, we appreciate your concern. Now please, explain the process and options. I'm all ears. Short of that, give us some breathing room."

"She's about to die."

"Betty, what have I just asked you to do?"

"Let's not fight. I've seen these things. I know you love her, and she's feisty. That makes it worse, because if she doesn't die, she'll be left with nothing. You don't think I see who you are? I do. You're vital people. I love that. Please!"

Betty pauses for drama and another moment of knowing. I ask, "Left with nothing? You mean ... a drooler?"

"Yes. But her cognizance won't be affected. She'll know. She'll need round-the-clock care for everything, and she'll know." I control my breathing in the daze of nurse Betty's uppercut. I meet her eye to eye but can't speak. Maybe I'm too weak to take control and opt for the knife over Rachel's veto. Maybe I fear the years of guilt ahead if she dies on the table. But I don't think so. Some stories are told without the narrator knowing where the story is headed. Looking back at this juncture is no different than living this juncture. Neither death nor fear is at issue here. It's information and dignity. Of course more is known in hindsight, because nobody would take a minute for dialogue at the time. We are left in the dark, as if the dark is where we belong. So, I stand pat. "Why can't you tell me our options, or what comes next?"

Nurse Betty listens benignly. She sees and drifts off, shaking her head.

I'm beside myself with uncertainty. I can easily defend my mate against the urgent needs of nurses and the youthful ambition of a surgeon whose speech impediment may indicate cranial pressure, possibly subarachnoid. But I feel increasingly defenseless against the phantom. It grows and populates around me. I can't breathe in here, which makes this place a perfect culture for darkness and fear. Evil loves a vacuum. This I know.

My mate is now pierced with steel needles at six or eight places on her body, and her greatest concern so far is for her hair. I will not question her rationale, because I can't, because I shouldn't, because we share the greatest trust, which is trusting our lives to each other. So I won't yet question her mind, but I prepare to take over. The dark spirit moves the ball down the field at will. We are taking a pounding here. I don't know how long I can or should fend them off. Worried about her hair? That's crazy.

Maybe my confidence and belief are challenged more than those of my mate. I feel a tickle in my soul, call it growing doubt on her mental stability, that which I ardently defend. She touches the left side of her head now; is this a gesture of fear for the imminent loss of hair, or is she soothing a deep ache? She mumbles over our quick departure from this place and the many fine draughts awaiting and the importance of doing what you so look forward to doing and corned beef for me. Surgery? Are you out of your mind? Surgery is for those with no alternative, and we have proven ourselves apart from that.

She looks up at me. "I hate this. I just hate it."

"Me too," I assure her.

"I don't know why we're doing this. I'm not having surgery. I feel fine. Besides, I wouldn't have surgery anyway." I must consider her wishes, her values, her rationale, and I fairly succeed, until she blurts, "They want to shave my head!" I think she fails to recognize the gravity upon us. I'm thinking three plays ahead now, can't help it; perception spirals downward as swift and steep as a fall through the looking glass. We are half empty. I try the invasive scenario on for size. Let's say she's irrational, then what? I'll tell you what; a brain surgery could be authorized by me, and death or debilitation may result. But what if she's rational? What if mean old Mr. Death is only toying with our natural rhythm? My skin crawls with prospects for wrong judgment. I wish we could fast forward into next week.

Out of infusion CAT scan we descend again to the front. Rachel now shows increasing wear and tear. Is this the result of brow beating and iodine injected to her brain? Or is the bleed increasing pressure on her speech center? Her eyes glaze with a weariness I've never seen in her.

She shakes her head.

I tell her we may stay the night. She shakes again. I tell her that if she ever trusted anyone, she should trust me now. I tell her we're together and I've never felt stronger or clearer or more ready to make the right call.

"Play it somewhere else," she says, and I smile. I'm proud of her vigor so clearly sustained in the face of very long odds. But I plead for help and tell her that I can't fight her and the knives at the same time.

"So? Who's fighting? What do we need to stay for? You don't need to stay. What do I need to stay for?"

"For observation. Listen! They want me to take authority away from you. They want me to consent to surgery. I said I wouldn't do that. And I won't. But you have to help me. Please, help me. I think.... I think we need the results of the infusion CAT scan—"

"I already had a scat thing!"

"Yes. You've had two of them."

"I had two?"

Oy.

"Yes. We need the results of the one you just had."

"That was a scat thing? It was . . . different."

"Yes. This machine is more sophisticated. More information. We need that. I'll tell you something else. We may need the angiogram too."

Anthony pushes the gurney. He interrupts here—"Oh, you'll need the angiogram. They got to have that." Even those you think are different here let you know sooner or later that they're part of the same process. We've been pressured toward an unspoken inevitability now for five hours without five minutes of privacy or reasonable explanation.

"Ohh . . . ." she whines.

"Listen. I need some time. I need to make some calls. I need more data so I can make some decisions. But I don't know who to call. Who can I call?"

"I don't know. We need to get closed from here. If we can be closed I can froth this . . . thing."

"Okay. But not yet. We need to stay the night—"

"Why! I don't want to."

"Because I'm scared. I'm very scared, dear. You don't believe these people, and I don't know what to believe. But you have had a massive cerebral hemorrhage. We can't leave. I can't leave. You can't leave if you might go off. We don't know that you won't."

"Where would I go?"

"I don't mean you! I mean the bubble in your brain. Kablooey. Capiche?"

She looks glum. She pouts. Anthony wheels the gurney back into place in the central arena and draws a curtain around us for the idea of privacy, leaving us to our domestic squabble, which is all it is. Anyone here can tell you that; it's natural, they would say, a predictable result of the tension and deathly potential. We're alone for moments when the worst knife yet slices my heart; she cries, not in heaving sobs but in simple emission of tears. "I really don't like this one bit," she says. "I really want to leave here, and you're not helping me."

"Please forgive me. I know I may be doing the wrong thing, but I hope to correct myself as soon as I can. I need a little time. That's all. And I need your help for tonight. Just tonight. Please. I need to make some calls. Please."

An Indian woman enters our curtained space, as many people will, by whisking the curtain back and stepping forward. How can you knock on a curtain? And who has time for common courtesy anyway? No, we must press on; privacy is expendable, and the feeling is that dignity is equally discounted here, with far greater urgency at hand. This woman does not wear a red dot on her forehead but has dark, bright eyes, a complexion to match and a pronounced nose. She's younger than we are, but not by much. "Hello. I'm Dr. Visnawara. Will you please squeeze my fingers?"

Four others follow her in, specialists, perhaps. But they say nothing. They circle the gurney and stand there half-smiling like cherubic attendants. Rachel makes her wince with a finger squeeze and recites the month, the day, the year and the name of the President of the United States of America.

Dr. Visnawara smiles and makes a note. She touches Rachel's head, front and center, and draws her finger around to the left side and down in what feels like a trauma-center rendition of the consigliori's kiss. Pardon me, but her frigid ambience is palpable. She smiles with practiced confidence approaching bliss, and though we wait for an elaboration on this personal contact, the bliss is all we get. This touch of a learned finger lingers like a wet spot in a breeze, chilling. After an agonizing interlude of presumptive silence, Dr. Visnawara says, "We need the angiogram. I think you'll do fine. This does not look to me like a complicated procedure. We do this all the time, you know. All the time. Straight in." She scissors two fingers of her right hand—straight in. "We think you do not have a tumor. We think your vital signs are very good."

"You think that because I sold you five years ago. I don't want my hair shreaved."

"Oh, don't worry. It will grow back. Oh, you will do very good, I think. Very very good. I must tell you that you do have a chance of dying, but you also had a chance of dying yesterday and today, and you did very good on those. You must also know that we sometimes have morbidity on these procedures. But that is much better than dying. And I think you have done very good so far. So maybe you will do good tomorrow."

"What's tomorrow?"

"We must have surgery tomorrow. We should have surgery tonight, but we're very busy now, and you are doing all right, and we need the angiogram before surgery, so, tomorrow. All right? Good night?"

"Wait a minute," I say. "We've only heard about the surgery in oblique reference. Nobody has told us about the surgery or the options. We haven't yet decided that we want surgery."

"But you must. Otherwise she will surely die. Five percent per year. Twenty years. You have been told this. We have it on your chart. I must go now. Someone else will be around to answer your questions tomorrow." She leaves to meet her busy schedule. The entourage files out like goslings as I realize we've been disclaimed, legally, before witnesses.

"But we haven't agreed!"

Rachel is about to cry, really cry, not so much with realization, I think, as frustration. They won't leave her alone, but they won't talk to her or recognize her. She is, to them, irrational, ostensibly vegetative. She still speaks, but the voice is not connected to the person in the legal sense. Unless of course someone might want to make a case. In that case, she has been read her rights, which are indeed greater than zero, evidenced by the place granted to her in the machination of the juggernaut. "Go away," she tells me. "I want to be alone."

We are surrounded again by agonizing distraction, audible and visible as a train wreck in slo-mo. I smile. I touch her arm. "I'll be back in five minutes."

I find the phone booth in the anteroom. I could use my cell phone but could never hear over the wailing and groaning. I could go outside, but that seems too far away for Rachel's interests. And the payphone inside does have a door that stifles the noise when it closes. I move slowly, stunned, bogged as a runner in a dream. I feel helplessness oozing from my pores. I am stuck on inertia and a stunned inability to take care of things. I could pee in my pants and fit right in. I'm at least cognizant of fundamental delamination, so I go to basics, wondering if I'm still rational. I must first control my breathing. I must dispel the dark spirit and chaos infusing the space around me. I want to yell. I think it might help scare the phantom, but I simply can't handle an arrest right now, even on a misdemeanor.

I rack my brain for a name of someone who might offer guidance but can think only of well-intentioned friends who would offer solace, sympathy and assistance. Finally, after several long minutes, I recognize brain lock—that mode of mental shutdown in which the mind seeks the obvious solution but can't find it any more than a fly can fly through a windshield because it's a fucking fly and insists on the most visible route, banging into the glass straight ahead over and over again because it can so plainly see the life waiting on the other side, till it finally exhausts itself, drops, rolls over and dies on the dashboard. Only those flies with composure and the intelligence to back off and look sideways have a chance to escape.

Fucking flies.

So I back off and go to low idle, seeking calmness, only calmness, allowing all thoughts to fly away, sideways as it were.

Once calmed, breathing slowly with the mental lockup unlocked, the feeling changes. I wait for direction if not guidance, but like a diver at depth in the dark I can't tell up from down. I could pump a little air into my buoyancy compensator and let nature take its course, with its love letting me rise slower than my slowest bubbles to the surface—except that this place is out of my depth. I have no buoyancy compensation or coordinates beyond a phone booth in a trauma center. My confusion is real as the greasy surfaces and stale air surrounding me. I wonder if I look unhinged, if I'll be strapped to a gurney and rushed up for a scratch thing, to be sure.

The light reveals its access route suddenly, as it usually does: Hawaii, where more money is extracted from more believers than at the Vatican. Well, maybe not more than the Vatican, but Hawaii now spawns the biggest industry in who-do, foo foo, aerie faerie, wanna-be, sappy-ass fruitcake snake oil on the face of the earth. I discount it as the next phase of tourism.

Why then does it come to me?

Because the real item also resides in Hawaii. Modern times, population and greed have always spawned imitators of the genuine article. The real McCoy is now as rare as innocence in Times Square. But I know a woman there, Carol, my friend from Aikido. We trained together for years, throwing each other hither and yon. Her grasp of street-level reality does not inspire confidence; she too could be wheeled up to infusion scratch pan in a heartbeat. Yet she is familiar with the invisible world, its population, inclination and contact. She's psychic—the real item, one who can see the future but won't take a look because knowing in advance cannot change what will happen—it can only cause anxiety and then some, and then any normal people who find out will think her a loony. Besides that, each look leaves her wasted, ashen and beat for hours or days. I tell her it's just her period, but she has yet to laugh. She took a look for me once before. I don't know who else knows of her psychic skill other than she and I. She won't use it on anything less than dire circumstance, and here we are.

"Hey, Carol."

"Hey! You! I knew you'd call!"

"No you didn't. How could you know?"

"Well, I didn't know it would be you. But I stayed home from class tonight. First time in two years for a Wednesday night. I just couldn't go. What?"

"Hey, I hate to call you out of the blue with bad tidings. But I'm in a real jam. I need some guidance." So I debrief to a laywoman across an ocean. I'm careful with objectivity, profiling the aggressiveness here, the unequivocal certainty of surgery with no options as well as Rachel's chief fear, for her hair. When I finish, we wait. I hear her breathing and imagine her strange twitch, in which electricity in frightful voltage arcs the planes of being and knowing—not exactly like the scene in *The Bride of Frankenstein* where the kinky haired wife comes to life at the top of the tower during a thunderstorm with hellish lightning bolts searing the night sky. Carol's communion with the cosmos has much better effects and is more realistic.

Outside, the lament demands equal time. Carol too hears the muffled dirge, not as a distraction but as integral to the bigger picture, as part and parcel of the life force, in this vortex of transition and the chorus of humanity along for the ride.

In a minute Carol says, "Do the surgery. The hair will grow back."

"That simple?"

"I think so."

"But I . . . I need to get some information. Who do you know who deals with head stuff? Brain stuff?"

"Hmm . . ."

"How about Upledger?"

"Ooh! Yeah! They'd know! I need to call my girlfriends to get some numbers."

"I'm in a crush here."

"Twenty minutes. Okay!"

I walk back to the melee and meet Rachel on the way. She is rolling her wheeled monitor back from the bathroom. "They're pumping this stuff into me by the quarter. I had to pee."

Nurse Betty doesn't get physical but gives us the look of death, but by now we're used to it. So she says with threatening undertone, "You. Must not. Do that."

I tell Rachel I have some calls in to some alternative sources. We may have some outside guidance in a half-hour or so. In the meantime, we can continue to collect data here, ignore the noise and the scenery and the hard close. We'll plan to spend the night. By morning we should have a clear course. She wiggles on the gurney and says she's cold. She needs a blover. She doesn't respond to my situation report because she's weary or depressed or suffering cranial pressure, or all of the above.

I don't know much about Upledger, except that The Upledger Institute is commercially successful in its recruitment and training campaign. More importantly, the four or six people I know in Hawaii who have the ability to heal others with non-invasive means have all taken multiple training sessions in cranial-sacral therapy with Upledger. Seldom is heard a discouraging word; moreover, they hold the Upledger techniques in high regard. It's all I can think of right now.

In twenty minutes I call back. Carol gives me three names from Washington, Colorado and California, Upledger practitioners considered to be the very best. If they can't provide the necessary information, here is the direct number to The Upledger Institute.

The first number has been disconnected. A little girl answers the second number. She says she doesn't know when her mama will be home from her job. Mama is a waitress.

The third number is in Colorado. A soft-voiced man answers. He seems intelligent but can't hear for the wailing children and TV noise in the background—his background. He finally has the sense to take it in the next room. He listens and says he's not really trained in Upledger but in some other cockamamie discipline. He *thinks* we should *probably* go ahead and *consider* the surgery. Meanwhile, he'll do what he can from there.

From Colorado?

Up in the mountains?

I don't press him but thank him and check the clock; only nine hours to opening time at The Upledger Institute in Florida. I go back and tell Rachel we're on the right track, headed to the source; it won't be long now. She can't speak; whether for sadness or the other, I can't tell.

Her sister Sue arrives. A teenage boy in blue scrubs tells me that Sue is waiting out front but can't come back until I leave. I'll have to leave if Sue stays, because only one visitor at a time is allowed in the trauma ward. I ask him to please tell Sue to come back. I'll leave when she arrives. He rolls his eyes, like I've compromised regulations once more, and he leaves.

In a few seconds another young man enters in the white tunic indicating the higher, noncommittal echelon. His nametag says Phil. Phil reaches to put his fingers in Rachel's hands but she shoos him away and tells him to get a calendar and turn on CNN. Phil smiles good-naturedly and asks that Rachel please remember three words, ball, ring and wristwatch. Then he says we have excellent news. He pauses, apparently to allow our excitement to register. We wait, and finally he informs us that the infusion CAT scan revealed that the bleeding appears to be contained for now. Better yet, the staff has reason to believe there is no tumor. We share marginal relief, hearing that we have been spared two dire potentials that, until that moment, we'd been kept unaware of. We look glum, perhaps sharing as well the realization that we only broke even on two bits of good news. But best of all, he says, we're on the schedule for an angiogram at nine a.m. He has two consent forms ready for signature, which is required, "because we do have some mortality in angiogram."

"What? No morbidity?"

"Oh, that, too."

"Thank you, Phil. We'll deal with this later."

"Nine a.m.," he chirps on his way out. We share a moment of acceptance and progress. I touch Rachel softly as a means of assurance; things are looking up. I inhale to tell her that Sue has arrived. But then Phil dashes the curtain aside and swoops back in. "What were those three words?"

Rachel thinks.

"I have an idea," I say. "How about if you and Rachel both write them down, and we'll see who gets it right?"

"You know we're only doing our job here," Phil says.

"We don't mean to complain, Phil. But your job here seems to be an ongoing monitor of confusion in the patient. The irony is that the process has confused both the patient and me. Maybe I'm the control here, demonstrating that a non-hemorrhaged observer shares the confusion. I only want to keep this honest, Phil. I think whatever confusion is here is generated by this place and this process, which seems confusingly secretive and repetitive. Do you remember the words?"

Phil smiles briefly and exits. Rachel calls out, "Ball, uh . . . ring. And uh . . . uh . . . wristwatch!" But Phil is gone, perhaps to log evidence of confusion, paranoia and resistance on our chart.

Besides no privacy and constant, unannounced intrusion of visitors bearing good news and/or mortality disclosure, we are constrained from conversation beyond words or phrases barked from the foredeck to the cockpit in heavy weather. Like the noise of a gale or storm or hurricane, the lament is difficult to imagine. A new woman from the blue team swings the curtain aside. She spreads her legs, plants her feet, crosses her arms and tells us we still have a visitor waiting out front.

I go out and debrief for Sue: we think we have no tumor and they want an angiogram and surgery in the morning. Sue says in a heartbeat, "Well, that's terrific!" Sue does not share her sister's sense of the natural world. Sue's children take antibiotics like M&Ms, because they cure what ails you. If this were a scene of sisters reversed, Sue would be in pre-op already, thanking her lucky stars that a brilliant young doctor would soon cleave her head. I don't mind, for we each must allow the other to choose her beliefs. Terrific, however, this is not.

I remind her that the watchwords of the hour are calmness and assurance. Sue must know these things already, I think, but I warn her that she must not under any circumstance press forward on the side of the doctors. It will only compound resistance. We want nothing—Nothing!—through the night but neutrality. I will go in with her, and then I must leave, for the poor dogs have been in the car ten hours now. I will drop them off at the office in town after walking and watering them and bedding them down. Then I will return. She should stay with Rachel no matter who says what until I return. We must maintain our vigilant guard against heroism.

"Heroism?"

"That's when they cut you up for your own good."

"But she needs the surgery!"

"Sue. Please. We need a holding pattern until sunrise. Please."

Sue gives me a few sheets of paper, a printout on subarachnoid hemorrhage she pulled off the Internet. I stash these pages in my pocket, and we go in together.

I remind Rachel that the bleeding is contained for now, and she has no tumor. She laughs short. I tell her I will take the dogs and be back to spend the night. I write my cell phone and office numbers in six-inch letters on her folder that is already a half-inch thick. She says fine, but if she calls and I'm not around she'll take a cab. She gets up to use the bathroom again. The blue team responds like the secret service to a loony with a gun.

Knowing Rachel as congenial to a fault, I assess this scene, as the blue team cannot. She is simply distressed and has to pee, but to them she's a wacko who won't cooperate and who has a shrill complaint. "Get away from me!" All they want to do is help, and all she does is resist, or so it seems.

I take my leave in a blush of expedience. I need out. I see my opening and make my move, leaving my mate behind. I tell myself I must stay strong, that engaging the mind is the best cure for motion sickness, that I should tend to details in order to improve the big picture. But the truth here too is harsh; the air outside is oxygenated and ion-charged instead of stifling, overbearing and death scented. Yet the scene is also boisterous, noxious and disturbing, with the medivac helicopter landing just across the drive.

This is not the old familiar helicopter of Hawaii tourism and Magnum, P.I. That was the Bell Ranger 500 helicopter, scorned by those people who live under the fly zones, because they sound like giant mosquitoes. This is the full-bore Apache attack unit dreaded by the Afghans, Albanians and anyone else who dares to fuck with these colors don't run. A sixty-foot rotor span over flashing reds and blues and focused beacons scanning for escapees make this beast outshine a lighthouse at Christmas, out-rumble Godzilla. The downdraft gusts to ninety knots. Cinders whip sideways, irritating my eyes and stinging my face. The yelling and arm waving looks like an attempt to orchestrate the monstrous rotors and the *Whomp! Whomp! Whomp! Whomp! Whomp!*

We have endured for most of a day and a night the mutterings of *crazy, insane, idiotic, irrational, some people,* and on and on. Yet in the piercing cinders and hot gusts I am affirmed by the ambulance screaming in unison with the screaming chopper, as I watch a victim who couldn't say no or forgot to politely decline. The patient is hustled from one thrill ride to another, chopper to gurney to ambulance. The patient is as wired and plugged as Rachel, its hands gripping the gurney sides, its knuckles white. The ambulance gets scratch in a gratuitous display of drag strip urgency or the finest medical services insurance money can buy. Or military might, or something or other. Or maybe it's only youthful exuberance, the kids trying to find out what this bucket can do. The ambulance doesn't make third gear, because it's only fifty yards to the door, which is obviously too far to walk or ride on a gurney, and it bills out for seven hundred more dollars.

I turn my back on this DMZ and walk quickly in long strides, stretching it out, planning my schedule on the way. A nonstop hour later the car has repeatedly reminded me of its needs. The dogs are walked, peed, watered and bedded down in my office. I need a beer or some wine, but I can't. I feel bad and out of control, as if life is rolling its eyes up into my head.

I know from heavy weather at sea that the sickness is best fended off by activity. I fetch the printout Sue gave me and skim the fundamentals, what the hospital staff seems unwilling to convey for fear it could be misconstrued and followed by litigation, or misrepresented and followed by litigation, or misdirected, wrongly applied or inaccurately repeated, followed by litigation. I had folded these pages into quarters but then wonder why I did that, when thirds would have fit so much better in my inside pocket. So I unfold the quarters and refold in thirds, making progress all the time.

Molly and Dino are settled now, but they'll need to eat and pee near sunrise and given a chance to take a dump outdoors. I go downstairs for a chat with Sebastian, the night-shift doorman. Doormen or doorwomen or even doorpersons seem unnecessary, except as egregious proof of security, though it's only a concept to benefit those who need reassurance. I like opening my own doors, and the door staff would be hard pressed to interfere with a serious intruder, but the door staff is generally alert. Sebastian is a kid from Cameroon; no speaka too gooda de English, but he's a smart kid with good manners. He listens and nods. He cannot be walking dogs while he is working. But he is off in the morning at seven and can walk them then, if that will do.

It will be perfect, I tell him, so we go up together for introductions; so Molly won't maim him for breaking and entering. The dogs take to Sebastian, and I review breakfast, which is dog food in a bag, in case they don't have that sort of thing in Cameroon. Sebastian grants me a tolerant smile, so I show him how to fill their water dish and outline the basics of a short walk just across the street so they can pee. And maybe take a dump.

"A what?"

"A dump. A shit. You know . . ." I hunch my back, grunt and blow raspberries. Molly loves this. Eyebrows and concern overarch Sebastian's patient smile. I slip him twenty bucks, the universal muscle relaxant. We say goodnight, shake hands, he leaves, and I gather my things.

But my skin jumps when the phone rings. Nurse Betty is on the line to tell me the angiogram will be in the morning, and consent forms must be signed. In the meantime, Rachel has been moved out of the ER and officially admitted to the hospital. She's in Nine West, Intensive

Care. All her clothing, her purse and wallet were removed to the vault for safekeeping. I can process forms for reclaiming them tomorrow.

"Can you get me a cot, please? I'm staying with her."

"No. You can't. Not in Intensive Care. It's highly infectious. Besides we don't allow family to stay in rooms. Not in this hospital."

"Highly infectious?"

"We have no beds in the Neurology ICU. She's in the Pediatric/ Burn ICU."

"Great."

"She's doing fine and getting very good care."

"No surgery in the middle of the night?"

"We hope not. I have both your phone numbers. I'll make sure her night nurse gets them." She gives me the direct number to Nine West and says, "I have to tell you again, she has all the classic symptoms of memory loss and speech loss."

"Betty. I don't doubt your assessment or your intention. But you have no base of comparison. She's always been that way. Her hero in life is Lucy . . . . That's *I Love Lucy*."

"I know who Lucy is."

"Good. Did you think Lucy had an aneurism? Nobody said Lucy had an aneurysm." I pause for comprehension but get only exasperation. Nurse Betty sighs into the phone. "Did you ever notice young Dr. Michael speaks with a heavy lip?" She laughs. "What's that? Has he had a CAT scan?"

"I'll let you go now. Try to get some sleep."

"Where's Sue?"

"You mean the sister? She went home. Good night."

I sit and stare. Molly and Dino are up again; our routine does not account for so much going and coming and strange people at all hours and phone calls. And they want to know what's up with the tension, so thick you could choke on it.

Highly infectious?

And where's the alpha bitch?

Thank God for dogs. They know but can't fill in the details, so I tell them. They cry and nudge. We commiserate, and I gain marginal comfort. I lie down in my clothing and feel drowned and dredged. Numbness is stunning and overwhelming, like what comes between impact and pain. I get up, drink a beer and consider puking. I lie down and watch the spinning room; you don't have to be drunk to have it spin on you.

I sit up and lie down and get up to call Sebastian and tell him we're covered. "Covered?"

"I'm staying. I'll walk the dogs."

"And maybe take a dump. Okay."

"Thank you, anyway."

"Okay."

I lie back once more and begin the sorting process, the nervously energetic drive of humans unable to achieve adequate calmness, in the belief that thinking a thing through over and over will ease the mental muscles into perfect, happy sense. The imagery of a dark spirit and wrestling match between it and me crosses my mind but is banished, or in modern terms repressed, for its arcane, foolish, fearful nature. Which of course is the perfect entrée for the shadowy one, who comes on in formidable mass, not anthropomorphic, not with limbs and a cape like Darth Vader or clashing plaids like the Joker. This spirit is again aligned with what I've learned, seen and felt. To imagine that the ether is not populated is naïve. Then again, I can hardly call my nemesis an individual; it's so amorphous, unwieldy, rank and pervasive. I want to grasp and beat him and send him on his way, which of course is another simplistic motivation born of our yen for convenience.

I can't, yet I can engage him:

I don't know who you are, why you came or where from, but I dare you to come forward now.

I watch the clock pass two and ease on down to four. I don't care.

I control my breathing with long, deep draughts, and I conjure those images that seemed fundamental to the healing crisis of our past. I've sensed a mystical connection since childhood between the little fishes and myself. Call me introverted, antisocial, misanthropic, a gill-breather at heart. I'm most comfortable among cold-blooded creatures of garish color and innocent intent, whose daily lives revolve around predation, procreation and protection of territory.

I wish my needs were that simple and perhaps act out that simplicity in my thoughts. I knew Rachel shared my natural attraction to the sibilant depths but never so much as the day before the milestone mammogram, six months after her breast-cancer diagnosis. By then all her friends and acquaintances and doctors wished her well with sad resignation and common recognition that the end was near. She had declined "the great cures" in lieu of "the easy way out." So thorough was consensus that she asked if it made sense to me, dropping thirteen percent of her body weight, drinking vinegar and stinky juice, popping enough vitamins to give Babar a kidney stone. "Am I crazy?"

"Of course you are," I assured her every time. "What does that have to do with anything?" The six-month mammogram was scheduled for a Monday and loomed no less gray and sinister than a swim off the beach under gathering clouds at dusk, as if a carnivorous phantom lurked there. Shark imagery most often conjures fear unfairly. We'd met many sharks in our marine lives and knew that sharks are no big deal beyond the mutual sniff, assessment and exchange of curiosities. But we were afraid, in need of a diversion, so we decided on a reef outing for Sunday, the day before the telltale test.

Two reefs on Maui enjoy adequate protection from the human onslaught, classified as Marine Life Conservation Districts—no anchors, no boats or boating traffic and no fishing, including hooks, nets or spears. Ahihi Bay is on the south end and Honolua Bay is up north. We chose Honolua, even though the north swell is often up through late spring, and on Sunday the place would likely be packed with people. We hadn't been there through the winter and wanted something fresh, never mind the swell off the ocean or the crowds; we'd go way out, beyond the masses and shore break.

But the parking lot up by the road was empty, and we hiked down to an empty cove. The bay was flat as water in a bowl, and though we noted these strange conditions, we didn't call them eerie—we didn't remark on them or say anything. We were out for recreation, not assessments of strangeness. We wanted away from strangeness. We welcomed the same silence above the surface that we would find below.

In the water in a minute, we cruised easily out a hundred yards or so. With no wind, no surge and no humans, visibility below seemed as clear as above. In a short distance we were joined by six or eight raccoon butterflyfish, perfect little beauties whose masks rippled back from their eyes into a radiant yellow. Then came forty or fifty yellow tangs in radiant yellow with no ripples. A few dozen Moorish idols and parrotfish came in with many wrasses, reef triggerfish, fantail filefish and three-foot trumpets in both silver and yellow. The puffers came in pairs, spotted, blue and gold and boxfish hovering among the Hawaiian lionfish (very rare in open water), angelfish, damsels, black durgons, pinktail durgons rarely seen so shallow, a spotted eagle ray, a few ulua, some unicorns and a school of goatfish.

You get the picture: dozens and then hundreds and soon thousands of fish in waves of color, innocence, curiosity and something else, converging slowly from all points to hover in a circle of light and shimmering, spectral color. Fish don't wear smiley faces but use their lateral lines to emit neurons, in this case neurons of well-being and assurance, at that moment neurons in unison and with ample amperage to convey their message. They hovered and watched the center of their gathering, which was us.

Rachel came up crying her eyes out. I trembled in the presence of God, telling us we were covered by whatever magic ever existed in heaven and earth, and don't forget the deep blue sea; it would be all right. We hugged in a brief, easy tread and had no more doubt through the following day. The all clear came by dusk on Monday like another shark, perhaps, an animal spirit passing through. Meanwhile, on that Sunday morning, we dove back down to celebrate with our friends. It was the crowning contact of our life under water.

So I dive again, seeking the little fish in the depths of my straining dream on the ninth floor in downtown Seattle. I want that feeling again, but it won't come at will or by desire or for personal need. I reckon sleep at about four-thirty, when images merge and patterns of fact and number swirl asymmetrically, lose their color and go deep. Light fades. A hospital monitor would show rapid eye movement as a great frayed net sweeps the reef to capture the magic for removal to aquarium display far, far away, so that the people may be educated and the children amused—*No! No! No! You can't do that!*

Oh, but it must be done, cries the needful voice. I watch in horror. The net is a fine mesh made of thin, invisible nylon and catches every speck of life and color and light—even the plankton cling to it, for such is the power of the dark spirit moving over all of all, having its way, a juggernaut of disastrous need. I cry out but have no voice until fatigue turns my silent cry to a whimper and a twitch, and desire takes a rest.

A long time later, from the abyss of what feels like the waters of forgetfulness, a little talk-bubble rises. I can see the words inside all jumbled up. We rise, gaining momentum, nearing the surface and then breaking it, bolting up and bursting out: *Wait a minute! If odds are running five percent annually, you're still looking at five percent each year whether you go twenty years or a million! Waiiiit!*

6

———◆◆———

You're Doing So Many Things to Upset Us

The haze solidifies when the phone rings. "Mmnnguh."

"Is this Rachel's husband?"

"Nyuh."

"You need to get down here right away."

I bolt again like a bit player in *Night of the Living Dead*. Didn't I do that just a second ago? Have I slept at all? "Wha? Wha's it? Wha's wrong?"

"Your wife is leaving."

"Leaving?"

"She's disconnecting herself. She says she's leaving."

"Ohhh . . . Put her on."

"Okay."

Oh, God.

"Hello, dear."

"What are you doing?"

"I'm leaving. Can you pick me up? I need my clothes. They stole my clothes and my horse and everything. These people are so rude."

"Rude?"

"Yes. The nurse last night was horrible. What a mean man. I finally told him I didn't even like him. You know what he said? He said, 'That's okay. I don't like you either.' I've had it. Then the Indian bitch comes in this morning and starts yelling at me. I don't need that."

"Yelling at you? About what?"

"About all my questions. They won't even answer my questions. She yelled at me because I asked the same things last night. She says, 'I already told you about that and I'm not wasting any more time on you.' What a cunt."

Rachel uses the C-word as often as she takes aspirin. I think these women have failed in patience and respect. I'm partial to Rachel, because the doctor should be more flexible to the needs of patients in the throes of subarachnoid pressure. Yes, Rachel can be demanding, like now. So what?

More importantly, I sense new hazard, new symptoms of delusion. We may have a theft, a mean nurse and a spiteful doctor, but her complaint goes murky when she accuses the staff of switching pictures on her.

"Those aren't my pictures! They won't even slide me my pictures! I don't think they even have them!"

"I don't know what you're talking about. What pictures do you mean?"

"My x-ray pictures. They won't sl . . . sl . . .

"They won't show you?"

"Yeah. They won't show me. They showed me somebody else. It didn't even have my name on the thing."

Oy. We know that calamity and death in hospitals can and does result from clerical error. Yet I fear the other phantom here. She is demanding film negatives from the morning angiogram, and they have not come forth. They gave her Valium, she says, and then refused to share the results.

"How do you know it was Valium?"

"I don't know. But they gave me something so I couldn't even . . . you know." She knows as well that the brain appearing on the monitor wasn't hers.

"How do you know it wasn't yours?"

"It didn't even have my name on it."

"Oh." I don't press here. I don't ask if she thinks it was stock footage on the monitor, or if they maybe had a shill plugged in one room over, a certain goner they keep on hand to close tough deals like this one.

I feel the odds growing against her logic; did she expect to see her name stamped on her brain? Or was another name printed at the bottom of the screen? "How do you know they gave you a drug?"

"I felt it. It wasn't like the dots or the other. They put it in my veins. They said the angiogram would be real painful, you know, right in here."

"I can't see you, dear."

"Right here, up to my ribs, and then it wouldn't hurt. But I got real fuzzled and didn't know what was going on. I know it's not right."

"I'll be right down."

"I'm leaving."

We are known by now as the troublesome two who won't go along. As the trauma center for five states, this hospital deals in tremendous volume with equal pressure that keeps staff fuses as short as our own. We ask questions and have yet to display gratitude. I will overhear and be told through the morning that surgery should have been last night, and now the whole staff is upset because we declined. Now Rachel could die and I mean right now, and it's our fault. Except that first, before dropping dead, Rachel is leaving.

"Look. Please! Do me a favor. Stay put till I get there. I need to run the dogs out for a whiz. I have to whiz and brush my teeth. Wait. I'll be there in twenty minutes. Please relax until I get there."

"I have to! They took my drawdles! Hurry up. And bring me some lipstick!"

Off her fricking rocker. I bolt again and crunch gears, my own brain smoking at dangerously high rpm. Yet I'm gratified by small efficiency. I serendipitously save two minutes by pissing along with the dogs instead of treating it as separate functions of species. With a half-minute shower to wake me, I'm out the door nine minutes after the call.

But I'm right back in. It's nearly ten a.m. in Florida. I call The Upledger Institute. Dazed and stressed, I explain my urgent need for guidance. The woman at the other end doesn't know where Dr. Upledger is right now, but he's in the country; in fact he's in town and should be found in the next hour. Dr. Upledger? The Pope, himself? "Perfect." I give her my cell number and the number in the room, where I'll be in a few minutes. Which I am in seven minutes, after clearing customs.

Anonymous staff follows me into the room to ask for a finger squeeze, the date and the name of the President of the United States of America. They probe at will. One of them says, "Don't stand there, please." I step aside. They make notes and leave with no further discussion.

At least things are calmer now. A man in a white tunic with less hair than me attends Rachel. He says hello. His name is Lawrence. His handshake and demeanor seem reasonable and stable, and he has not scratched out his nametag in favor of a hand-hewn *Larry*. Beneath his name is *Head Surgeon*.

Lawrence has not seen the sun in recent months, nor does he appear physically fit, but he's physically intact and conveys a fortitude, stability and social skill hitherto lacking in hospital personnel. I ask why Rachel was so upset this morning with the Doctor who appears to be from India.

"That would be Dr. Visnawara."

"Yes. Rachel feels this woman is of the Cuntish sect, and I have to tell you we don't mind Sikhs or Kurds, but we cannot allow any Cunts."

He won't smile but says, "We're all under pressure here. We want to resolve this soon. I'm here to answer questions."

The phone rings. I know who it is. Rachel asks about the slice he wants to make in her melon. "Hello?"

"Hello. This is John Upledger . . ."

John Upledger is the most highly regarded purveyor of non-western remedy for cranial-sacral injury in the world. His name is generic. Having him on the line is like speaking to, say, John Kleenex or John Xerox or John Pepsi or John General Motors. It's all relative to personal values, of course. But I ask him to hold, please, so maybe he can talk directly with the surgeon. We can save time that way, dispensing with me, the messenger. Dr. Upledger says all right, and I announce with a degree of exoneration, "I have John Upledger on the line."

"Listen," Lawrence the neurosurgeon says. "I only have a minute here. If you could take that call later it might be best. Okay, we make the incision here, behind your ear and run it up in a horseshoe shape up to here, where you part your hair. About nine inches . . ."

"Yes. Sorry, Doctor Upledger. I thought the neurosurgeon might want to, you know. But . . ."

"I know."

"It's an aneurysm that bled but it didn't blow out. The infusion CAT scan showed the bleeding is contained for now, but the clot is big; they're saying four centimeters. Oh, and no tumor. I don't know what to do. We don't belong here. They're coming at us like a tidal wave. We have a history of breast cancer with a complete cure with no surgery, no radiation and no chemotherapy. Nobody here will tell us if we might—"

"Listen," Upledger interrupts. He waits for a settling moment. "I know what you're going through and what you're hoping for. I know what they're putting you through. I know they're urgent and insistent and keep you ignorant. I know they're refusing to talk to you or explain the basics. But I have to tell you, sometimes we have to depend on these fellows for a few things we have no alternative for, not yet, and this is one of those times. You simply have no choice here. You must proceed." He is done. He waits for comprehension.

"I understand. It's that simple. It's cut and dried. Thank you. At least hearing it from someone from our school makes the decision easier for me."

"This may be a small consolation for now, but I can tell you, this is a straightforward procedure for these guys. You have no choice. There is nothing else we can do for a subarachnoid bleed. Nothing. I'm sorry."

"I understand. I appreciate your help."

"Good luck to you and your wife."

"Thanks." I'm off the phone and back in the world of intense caring.

"No," says Lawrence the neurosurgeon. "I'll stop short of your hairline. You won't see it. I mean, you'll see it for a few months, but not after the hair grows back. We don't remove your scalp. We fold it back. We cut a section from your skull. We lift the lobe of your brain and remove the clot. Time is critical. You're already at forty hours or so. At seventy-two hours the clot breaks down. Many vessels in your brain will constrict. You'll spasm and stroke. Once we clear the clot, we clip the aneurysm."

"Clip it?"

"With a small titanium clip. It stays in forever."

"Then you skull my hat back?"

"Yes. We secure that section with two titanium plates. Small ones that won't set off security alarms."

She lays back and sighs, "That's crazy."

He nods and moves to the counter at the end of the room to make notes in Rachel's folder. "That was John Upledger on the phone," I tell her.

"Who's he?"

"He's the pope of alternative cranial-sacral remedy. He says we have no choice. We must have the surgery." She sighs again. "I'm not going against you," I say. "I'm only telling you my own, personal position. My standard is what I would choose for myself. I think surgery is not a clean choice. We may see complications. But avoiding the surgery is a dirtier choice. We can't do that."

"I can do that."

"There is no alternative source. John Upledger says we're dealing with internal pressure. There is no other remedy attempted anywhere." Her lips tighten. She smiles to hold back the tears. "If I was you, I would hate having surgery, because I want to have a spiritual death at home, not in this insane asylum. But I think we have a chance at success and many more years of life and fun. I can't give up that chance, not for a spiritual death right now. I can't."

I move to the counter and tell Lawrence lowly, "We want to schedule this."

"You're making the right choice. Believe me." He is walking out before this sentence is finished. I walk alongside, willing to accompany him all the way to his house if necessary to complete this session.

"You understand, I hope, that we come from a completely different belief system. I want to help facilitate the surgery, but I can't do it alone. Please don't assign the Indian woman to us. And if you wouldn't mind, any disclosures on death and morbidity can be made to me. Not to Rachel. All right?"

"I'll do my best."

"Oh, and she's really upset about having her head shaved. Can't you lie? Tell her it's only a two-inch incision?"

He stops and stares at me in gentle disbelief, as if I'm nuts, as if this could be the set-up he's anticipated all along. "We don't mean to get anyone upset."

"I know that. But her stress levels are extremely high."

"They'll get higher. But that's better than dying."

"She's not afraid of dying. Do you understand that?" He tries but apparently can't understand our view anymore than we can freely accept his good intention, mixed as it is with superiority and certainty. So I state our position precisely: "It's less than living that she fears." And I cringe at the words that come next. "Death is preferable to morbidity. We've been resistant till now, because only Dr. Upledger explained the certainty to us."

"You mean the fellow on the phone?"

"Yes."

"He must have explained it to you in terms that were acceptable to you."

"Well, yes. He did."

With a sanguine smile indicating familiarity with our perspective all along, Lawrence begins walking away. He turns his head back to talk over his shoulder. "We'll have another angiogram this morning with radioactive dye. It's the gold standard." He finds his stride.

I catch up and walk alongside. "Yes, we learned about the gold standard last night. But I . . . I have one more question. Please. I'll be brief."

He stops. "If you have five-percent odds on an event, and those odds renew annually, what are your odds on the event in twenty years?"

It's a long time since the head closer crunched the front-end numbers, but his instinct is tuned to trick questions. I see him thinking: Ah, ha! That repartee about explaining things in acceptable terms was not the set up; *this* is the set-up. Finally, he says, "I'm not sure I understand your question." He scans for motivation.

"Okay. Let's say you're at the track. You really need some money, so you pick a twenty-to-one shot. You lose, so you pick another horse in the next race with the same odds, same payout. Twenty to one. You keep losing all day and all week, and by Friday, you've lost a hundred times at twenty-to-one. So you make another bet, another twenty-to-one shot. What are your odds?"

He smiles clearly, picture resolving. He won't speak until the words line up defensibly. I help him along—"The odds are still twenty to one. Aren't they?"

He shakes his head slowly but won't address the front-end. "This isn't the track. I don't know how the numbers were presented to you. Our statistics don't reflect what we *think* will happen. They measure what *has* happened. Fact. Nobody sustains a subarachnoid hemorrhage and survives twenty years without the surgery."

I nod. He has effectively conceded the blunder of his staff and at the same time overruled me with rational explanation. It's all we've waited on for forty hours. I want to ask how the team can dive into a wholesale brain shuffle when the point people can't pass muster on Statistics 101. But this face-off is over. Ambient pressure is dire; I too am resolved and relieved. I defer to circumstance, miffed and frustrated by so much delay in filling our simple need with a brief exchange of straight talk.

He allows me an ounce of encouragement with a slap on the back. He says nothing, as in no more words coming from him, but he cracks a marginal smile, bringing home the point, which is that nothing else can be said. So I say, "I just . . ."

"I know," he says. "It's time to move on. Surgery tomorrow morning. Eleven."

He goes his way. I go mine, back to the curtained space. I tell Rachel that we're scheduled for tomorrow morning. She shakes her head very slowly and only an inch to either side, and I see another IV on the right side of her neck, a gang-valve with four leads on quarter-inch valves into a matching spike piercing her jugular. "I don't know about this," she says of things in general. "I don't like it. I can tell you right now I wouldn't do this if you didn't tell me to."

She's crying. I want to say something but it sticks in my throat. Two nurses sweep the curtain aside and step in to check the valves, to measure this and that and take notes. I ask about the neck cluster. They say it looks worse than it really is, because it's only a back-up system, mostly, that was put in place as long as they were tapping the jugular. The really important one right here, is a tiny tube that runs to the top of the heart, just in case, you know.

Their simplistic explanation again presumes two levels of comprehension on the ward, the elevated one and the one for street level. They need the small tube in place for several reasons, they concede. Like pumping adrenaline on a quick shot to the heart, just in case. Or like drawing off blood quickly, just in case.

I think staff assessment of patient needs may be as numbed as we are. They talk goo goo, as if we can only work a puzzle with big, rounded pieces, then they serve up some downside potential, cold. Of course we asked for it, but their biomechanical safety net sounds gruesome and severe, drawing blood off, dosing the heart muscle with adrenaline, both procedures indicated by death or near-death conditions. I think my complaint is for lack of nuance, what no trench in any war has ever enjoyed. But why would they say something like that in front of a woman so upset? I think it was not because I asked them to, but then it is. So we're all annoyed, so I ask, since we're on the subject of blood. Will we need some? Is this not the time to make sure we have some?

They say we won't need some, because this procedure doesn't call for blood. One nurse moves to the file cabinet for another form; as long as we're here, we might as well get this out of the way. It's the blood pool consent form. I scan it and ask what's the difference between using the blood pool and unprotected sex with the donors.

Oh, but it's not that way at all, because blood donors are screened, they say. They crumble in cross-examination; screening is an interview, a series of questions on sexual preference, sexual history, sexual habit, intravenous drug use and general health. The end. I shitchu not. Purity of the blood pool is further ensured by the requirement that no blood in the pool can be paid for but must be donated.

"I'm not signing that," Rachel says. "Are you nuts?"

The curtain whisks again on a small woman with a large smile who seems apologetic and silent, no offense. I think she's heard about us. Her eyes roll brightly over our little space as if seeking a place to light, and she chirps, "Hi! I'm Frannie! I'm your family liaison social worker. I'm here to help you with any problems you might have!"

I think we no longer have a problem, other than the obvious problem of being here, waiting for brain surgery. We've made the difficult decision, thanks to brief exchanges with Lawrence of Neurology and John Upledger three thousand miles away. We only have to process the time between now and post-op.

Frannie says, "I want you to know that your complaint has been duly noted."

"What complaint?"

"About Dr. Visnawara."

"We didn't file a complaint."

"I did," Rachel says.

I shrug. "Who's taking note of this problem?"

"The team," Frannie says,

"We appreciate your effort," I tell her. "We have no complaint against anyone. Dr. Visnawara upset Rachel, so we'll want to avoid further contact with her. Okay? We don't want to get Rachel upset again. Okay?"

Frannie nods quick as a two-stroke engine and begins writing.

Intercepting the first two nurses on their stealthy exit, I ask what is Rachel's blood type. They dissemble. They don't know. "You don't know? You take blood every hour. You must know." They shrug and say we won't need blood anyway; we'll take care of it later. I will later learn that Rachel is B negative, not the rarest in the book but hardly available, not from me or her sister or her parents.

They take their leave as Frannie finishes with her notes and perks up to see what else might ail us as the curtain sweeps again on a black man in a shiny, sky blue suit, who steps inside unannounced. He wears a matching tie in baby blue and carries a matching hat. His shirt is lemon yellow. I am reminded of the reef, but this man is *niele*, which is Hawaiian for nosy and intrusive rather than curious and innocent. His Louie-Armstrong eyes roll over the scene with as many teeth. His voice is also deep and graveled but instead of *What a wunnerful world this would be*, his lyric is somber. "How do you do? I *am* The Reverend Brown. I make my rounds here. You see?" He glances toward the next space over, behind another curtain, where a very large woman bemoans the imminent loss of her life. "I am here. How do you do?"

"We do fine," I tell him. "Thank you. And thank you for stopping by, Reverend Brown. Have a good day."

"Ah! I see . . ."

"Thanks again. Bye, now."

He nods in retreat, his smile shrinking and uncertain. Rachel ups the volume on the TV overhead where a rural woman is being interviewed on a FOX special on Presidential morality and what the country needs to do. The woman harks back to better, simpler times: "Ah tell ya what Ah thank is 'at we shouldn't oughta have one 'at's got no morals. Ah thank we oughta get one 'at has morals. At's what's wrong wif all ese dang politicians. 'Ey ain't got no morals! 'Ey jiss havin' sekshull relations with all they damn interns. It's enoughta mike me sick!" The studio audience whoops and cheers in wild appreciation. They hush while the rural woman sings a ballad about love and morals. Rachel mutes it because the Reverend Brown is gone, leaving us to our needs and morals in private.

Frannie excuses herself, and we're alone at last for a blessed moment. Rachel sighs, "I can't let them shave my head. He wants to slice half my scalp off. He wants to cut away my skull."

"You remember on TV a few weeks ago they had an ad for hair transplants, and I asked if I should get one, and you pounced on me?"

"I didn't pounce on you."

"Yes you did. You said, 'What's that about? That's so you can look good for the young ones. That's the only reason men do that.'"

"This isn't the same as that."

"So I thought about the young ones and figured maybe you were right. Maybe I'm only lusty. But they don't come on like they used to, and I realized that you're the one I love, because you'll love me back no matter what I look like. Won't you? So what's with the shaved head and titanium parts in your skull? What's that? I'll buy you a floppy hat."

"I don't want a floppy hat."

"Yeah, well, I don't want a floppy date, and I promise, if you don't forget about your goddamn hair, I'm going to get my head shaved."

"You won't have a scar."

"I'll get one at the party store, red and green with festers and oozes. We'll cruise."

"Please don't."

"I won't. You please don't too."

We share another silence with no place to go, until the curtain opens on the new nurse with fresh quart bags. "Oh," Rachel moans. The day nurse proceeds to change the bags. They say Potassium Chloride.

"It's Gatorade," I console.

"I have to pee."

The nurse reaches for the bedpan, but Rachel is up. "You can't do that," the nurse says.

"Do what?" Rachel asks, hiking her jammies at the sit-down.

I step out to preserve what privacy remains between us. My cell phone rings, and it's Sue, asking if Rachel wants to talk to their parents who live near San Francisco, who are eighty, who called last night and were told by Sue's daughter Katy that Sue was at the hospital to be with Rachel. I say no, not yet, because Rachel is only now coming to terms with the situation and herself. She should be ready to speak to her parents in a short while, but not just yet—Rachel is only hours from a craniotomy. This is not her call; it's mine. She needs time to absorb her schedule peacefully and thereby gain the ability to discuss it peacefully with her parents. At the current moment, only more anxiety would result from a dialogue. "Give it an hour or two. Okay?"

Back in the room the nurse admonishes us in general to try for more stillness. She knows Rachel feels fine, and frankly, by appearances, everything is fine. But these drugs need cooperation to be effective.

"What drugs?" we ask in unison.

"Dilantin, to protect against seizure. Nimodopin to protect against spasm." She says both seizure and/or spasm are likely now. We must be still. She leaves. I sense a more frank honesty now. It gains momentum as our prospects reveal themselves. Then again, maybe they need us fully informed on these details, these consequences of misbehavior. I sense this disclosure is mandatory, informing Rachel of her rights. I know I've established my own legal record of challenging every incidence of non-disclosure. They think me difficult. They mean only to do their jobs. I sense these things, and I also sense, unfortunately, that I'm correct.

Rachel sighs and says she has given the situation some careful thought and knows she'll be better prepared to process things in a few days, after a brief return home to square the animals and take care of a few loose ends and get some additional information, which she sure as heck can't get around here. I remind her that we were in direct contact with the Pope of alternative cranial-sacral therapy only a short while ago. "I don't know what other information you have in mind."

"I can't know what other information exists as long as I'm smothered in this place, surrounded by these aggressive, smothering people."

I tell her that Sue has made a valuable contribution by retrieving the information she hungers for. I tell her I have reviewed it, and the apparent danger now is not so much from additional bleeding, because she's strong as a horse. The danger and urgency now stem from the hemorrhage itself. I suspect the aneurysm has been present for years, possibly since birth, though it has enlarged over time, stretching its own walls thinner to the point of leakage. At least it didn't burst.

"So if the hemorrhage was there for a long time, how do we know I'm not perfectly capable of processing it? How do we know I didn't have a simple headache, and now they want to cut me open?"

I remind her that only the aneurysm may be old, that yes, it was likely there for years, and now it has leaked. "The hemorrhage is new. It shows up bright on the CAT scan. That means it's fresh; as it congeals it darkens. Then it clots. Then it breaks down. It's the decomposition of the blood clot that changes the chemistry inside your cranium, in your brain. The other blood vessels cringe in contact with an aging clot. Seventy-two hours is the critical time. The other vessels shut down. Then you die or stroke."

"Listen. I might go along with this. But I want to go home."

"Rachel. You bled forty-five hours ago. Do the math. You can't go home."

Well, I've chosen the wrong words myself, but I'm bound to stumble sooner or later. Once spoken, they can't be retracted, but I back up and try again. "Listen. If I could lie down there for you, I would. If I could go outside right now and fight twenty muggers to get you out of here, I'd do it."

She listens, but I'm having no effect against the last roundhouse punch, that she may never again go home. "Well, maybe not twenty. They'd kill me. But three. I'd take on three." She half-smiles. "I'm right here with you, and we both know you're stronger than me. You're the strongest person I know. Physically, emotionally. Except for your hair. That's a disappointment, your hair anxiety. But you're a hero otherwise. You may be my new hero for all time. Who'd a thunk it? I'm here and I'll be here."

Her half smile relaxes now as her face puffs up, and she says, "You know I want to be cremated."

I nod. "Yes. You've mentioned that. And spread over Apple Tree Cove, because it's a place you love."

"Only a little bit. Take most to Hawaii. I love Hawaii. Hawaii is my home." I nod again. She looks worried and says, "But if you move away you won't be near me."

"I'll figure it out. Okay? I want to get through this. Fast but slow. Slow but fast. I'm on guard. I'm pretty good at this sort of thing. You know?"

"I know. I just wish . . ."

"Sh. I know." I let our wishes and knowing drift like smoke but not too far. "Do you want to talk to your parents?"

"What for?"

I don't tell her that it's a good thing to tell your parents you love them or they did a good job or something or other if you know you might die tomorrow. I say instead, "I think they'll feel left out if you have surgery and don't talk to them first."

"I can't. They'll just be so upset. Why should I put them through that?"

"They know."

"You told them? Why did you tell them?"

"Katy told them." She looks glum again. "I'll ring them up. They want to talk to you."

She nods. "I have a headache."

I ring for the nurse. We wait. In five minutes I fetch the nurse and report the headache. The nurse asks how bad is the headache. Rachel says not too bad. The nurse needs a number. What kind of number? One through ten. One is mild. Ten is major. "I'd say a four."

"Not a five?" asks the nurse.

"Okay. Five. No, four."

The nurse records four on the chart and in the computer and dispenses two Tylenol, also recorded.

Her parents are sitting by the phone. I turn around and tell them everything is fine. They respond quickly that they will not talk to Rachel if I think that best. They will defer to my judgment. I assure them I only wanted to wait so acceptance of the surgery could have a chance to sink in. They assure me that she must have the surgery. I assure them that we're well aware of their convictions on this, but we needed a little more time to process our own convictions. I now share their opinion on the need for surgery, and so does Rachel, but the subject is still tender and would best be left untouched.

"Rachel may still think she's going home," I tell them. "Talking to family can generate a fuss, and we've had plenty. But now, well, maybe she understands. I can't be sure." They concur. I tell them we have proceeded to schedule the surgery.

They repeat together, "Well you have to have surgery!"

I remind them to stay as calm as they can, especially on the surgery issue. I turn back and hand off the phone. It's small talk mostly, about the expedience of modern medicine and the pesky bother of an aneurysm with a massive hemorrhage. They talk a few minutes on life and love, the weather, small crises at home and a few bargains that really can't be beat. Rachel bids farewell to her parents, assuring them that she loves them as always and that she sorely hopes to talk to them tomorrow. They ring off, and another bridge has been crossed.

For the first time we hold hands in resignation; the abyss must be leapt into. This will be easier for me, it would seem, but then it's not, for I blow no smoke on relative strength. I'm merely a pup beside a she-wolf who understands winterkill. But assessments of relative courage are also brief. The curtain opens again on a middle-aged man with an apology. "I'm sorry," he says. "Is this a good time?"

"No. This is not a good time," I assure him. "What do you want?"

"I'm Dr. Goldfarb. I'm a psychiatrist. Do you have a few minutes? I understand you have questions. I'd like to answer them for you and find out a little bit more about your concerns. Is that all right?"

Dr. Goldfarb is small in stature, with a presence you could call contrived. I sense a method to this meekness, developed as a professional tool. Goldfarb's non-threat has dynamic magnitude. I suspect issues here that warrant process and a sincere willingness to work through this thing with a reach inside for feelings. In hindsight Goldfarb frames up as an effective distraction; the moment casts him otherwise, as a sniveling nuisance.

He eases gently to the sitting position as I address our concern, as requested. That is, we went out for a few beers two days ago and now face brain surgery. My wife has been repeatedly injected and drugged with very little explanation. I ask him how hard it is to recognize people like us, who will not subscribe to a foreign regimen on pain of death. I tell him the staff seems rational, but the momentum is rough, maybe not like an inquisition, with satanic relations proven, but with similar pressure to confess. I tell him that we are processing a severe paucity of reasonable dialogue, and we only want a few answers and to participate in the decision making process before it happens, not while it's happening, which has been the woeful case—or worse, after it's happened.

"I have to tell you," he begins. "You're doing things that are making everyone here quite upset."

"Things? What things?"

"Like sitting up. Or walking to the bathroom. Don't you know these things can raise your blood pressure? Even little things like that can be traumatic."

"What do you call a medivac helicopter ride? A walk in the park?"

"Well, yes, I suppose that could be traumatic too, but those people are experts."

"You say that could be traumatic, but I sense an air of condescension here. Have you experienced the medivac helicopter?"

"I'm so sorry that came out wrong. I don't mean to condescend or to humor you. I apologize. I only meant that the helicopter crew are very experienced."

"Experience is not the issue. If someone dies in the helicopter, are these guys likely to admit that pressure change or turbulence was the cause of death?"

"I believe they would, if that was the case."

"Have they ever lost anyone to pressure change?"

"They have not."

"Bingo! Don't you get it?" He is now hurriedly taking notes, getting it, I'm afraid, in a context other than the one intended. Still, I pursue. "Do they know about volume exchange and pressure gradients and Eustachian tubes?"

"Well, I'm sure they do—"

"You're sure? That's presumptuous. You're coddling me again."

"Well, yes, it is. I mean . . . presumptuous. I'm so sorry. I don't mean to—"

"And what about that cunt from India who yelled at me because I asked too many questions?" This is from Rachel, which makes me laugh, because I can't help it.

"She yelled at you?"

"Oh, yeah. She said I was wasting everyone's time. She said I was a fool to worry about my hair, because it was coming off anyway, and don't worry, they save it in case the mortician needs it to make me look good."

"She said that?" I ask.

Rachel nods.

The shrink and I share a moment of disbelief. "What about that? It sounds on the surface like this doctor is bringing her own unresolved problems in here when we're trying to understand something."

"I'm sorry about that. Your complaint has already been filed."

"By whom?"

"By staff."

"Are we to presume that staff got the complaint right?"

"You're going to have to trust us. You know that, don't you?"

"I'm trying my best. In fact, I'm willing to give this hospital an A+ on technical proficiency. That's presumptuous too, but I want to go along. The problem is, you get an F on presentation. How can we feel good about this when we're surrounded by smiley-faced students assembled to witness the death and morbidity disclosures? Do you know how many times we've been assured that Rachel might die or go morbid in the next thirty minutes? This process is thick with legal defense that undermines our confidence. I think legal defense is procedural here and it derives from policy, which derives from politic. The political function of the AMA is to safeguard its members from legal action. That's fine. Who doesn't want to cover his own ass? We have been led to believe that something may go wrong and often does go wrong, but those things happen mostly to those people less healthy than us. We felt on arrival here that we'd be better off with alternative treatment, and for two more days we've felt correct in that assessment, because we could not get a case made otherwise. All we got was assumption, presumption and *tour de force*, until I got word from Florida. On the phone, from three thousand miles away. Before that, we were expected to accept all the products and services you have to sell here for our own good, because you say so. We got excellent service, but it felt like the bum's rush followed by death and morbidity. I'm sorry too, but that's not the nature of a healthy system. It's like knowing what kind of car you want to buy and having a good idea of where you want to buy it, and then you go down to the dealer, and the first thing the salesman says is, 'Okay, here it is, now give me a check.' What do you do, pay up? This isn't a car lot, is it? But you do have your customers by the short hairs. All we need is some straight talk, and look at you, taking notes on the most obvious truth in the world. Look up for Christ's sake. You don't need to write anything down. It's written on the walls! We don't have a problem. You do."

"And they want to shave my . . . thing. I mean, not my . . . thing. You know . . ."

The little fellow is taken aback by my emotional display and Rachel's blubbering, but he hardly slows his note taking. He nods vigorously, prompting for more. I have more, but the curtain opens on a Chinese woman, who enters saying she is Dr. Hsu. "I'n Dot-ta Shu. Speet Patorogy. I wou rike to talk witchou. Hokay?"

"Dr. Shu?" I ask. She nods. I ask, "S-H-U?"

"No. Ah H. Ah S. Ah U. Is ah Chinee, you know, so we sperr diffalent."

"Ah. Dr. Hsu."

"Uh, Doctor. Please forgive me, but I'm Dr. Goldfarb, and I'm conducting an interview here. Do you mind giving us, say, twenty minutes? Would that be okay with you?" I think Goldfarb is miffed, suffering interviewus interuptus, on the verge of witnessing my volcanic eruption with clinically historic and potentially legal significance, which could prove ironclad for the defense and put a feather in his cap with a possible promotion, perhaps, someday.

"Ah, yes. But ah, may be I stay just, ah, ten minute, ask question. Then I go, and you ploceed. Yes?"

"I need about twenty minutes here, Dr. Hsu." Goldfarb is up with bold assertion in a three-meter pace, one lap and back down. "Make that thirty minutes. All right?"

"Ah! Hokay. Thuhty minute. Fust I ask, ah, tell me, do you hab speet pahrem?" She addresses this question to Rachel.

"What?"

"Ah, do you hab speet pahrem?"

"Do I hab speet pahrem?"

"Speech problem, goddamn it. Do you have a speech problem?" I'm laughing, can't help it. Rachel laughs too, it's so rich and so clear.

"No," she says. "I don't think so. Do I sound bad?"

"Ah, no. No, no. I come back. Hokay."

She leaves, giving Goldfarb proper pause to reach inside his mental sensitivity for some sensitive mentality. "Tell me something." He strokes his chin and thinks. "Do you feel . . . Okay, scratch that. Do you think . . . Do you think that we . . ."

But the curtain is swept again. It feels routine now, on a small stage, like Vaudeville. What an act. But the new arrival is a relief to all parties; we tired of analysis so soon, and Goldfarb was so lost in the script. "Hi. I'm Rebecca Nimmins, patient liaison. You have some questions?"

"Yes, we do," Rachel says, and asks again what she's asked four times already, about the length and placement of the incision. Nurse Nimmins steps forward more slowly than the others who answered this question in the last two days. She has no witnesses. We like her movement and her smile.

"Excuse me, Nurse Nimmins. I'm trying to conduct an interview here. I need, say . . ."

"I'm so sorry," she says. "I was sent by Dr. Luze. He'll be here in five minutes and wants all their questions answered beforehand."

Goldfarb sighs.

"It's all right," I tell him. "We're done with the psychological profile."

"You're done?"

"Yes. This is a simple situation. We shared our view of it with you. You're the first one who's listened. Thank you. Now we're done."

"I see." He moves to make a note.

"Good."

"Excuse me just for a minute, but you know, I'm going to make a recommendation here." We wait. "I'm going to recommend two signatures on the surgical consent forms. You'll need to sign those, you know." He is addressing me.

"You haven't been listening, have you, Goldfarb? Here we are pissed off as bees in a bonnet, sharing our frustration with you, and all you can do is go along like you understand and then turn right around with more of the same. That's rude, which is much worse than condescending."

"I . . ." But he turns to Rachel. "I know this is very scary for you. This is horrifying for you—"

"Cut! Cut! Cut! Who do you think you are, standing here telling her she should be horrified? Do you know what you've just said? That's what I profiled for you as the source of our problem here. So what's the first thing you do but repeat the offense?"

"That's validation, Mister."

"That's masturbation, Mister. You want to come in here and tell her she's looking good and doing great, okay. You're welcome. But preprogramming for fear is exactly what's wrong here, and we won't accept it. Furthermore, we're already resigned to surgery, and frankly we felt better about it before you got here."

"Look, I want to continue this dialogue. I'm going to recommend two signatures."

"Dr. Goldfarb, are you now or have you ever been in contact with the legal department?"

"What does that have to do with anything?"

"You'll get one signature. That's all you need. I'll stay clear and apart. If you press me on this or come back with more horror, I'll sue. If the surgery isn't scheduled on time, I'll sue. If Rachel walks out of here without a surgery, I'll sue. Do you get the picture?"

"You're a very difficult man."

"Bingo." I turn to Nurse Nimmins, in whom I sense care giving of a different cut. "That's the thing about this place. You take Goldfarb and me, both students of human behavior, human drive and need. But if we met under different circumstance, I wouldn't want to sit down and have a beer with him. I wouldn't want to hear what he has to say, because it's all apology as prelude to further advantage. It's like all those years of medical school were spent learning strategy." I speak of Goldfarb in the third person because he's gone. I overhear him in the hall, on the phone, debriefing on profile and intent. He refers to her and him, speaking with the legal department, I think, but I don't care.

I'm right about Nurse Nimmins, who conveys all the time in the world, whatever it takes. She's been to Hawaii and has personal interests of her own. Moreover, she understands that a five-percent annual chance times a million years is still a five-percent annual chance. The error comes from those who compile the front-end statistics. She explains the part of the printout from the Columbia University Neurology Department that Sue pulled from the Internet. The meaning I took from it was that all those people declining the surgery, if they were Grade I or II, with coherence and consciousness intact and only mild speech impediment, actually faced only a one in five chance of mortality.

No, again, she explains; this paragraph actually reiterates in better terms the five-percent concept. It further relates to the first six weeks following the bleed, in which most mortality occurs.

She is with us twenty minutes when the curtain opens on a woman who strolls in with another entourage. They circle the gurney and smile blissfully. "I'm Theresa. Dr. Smythe." Theresa is early thirties but doesn't exercise. She will administer the anesthesia. Her face is sweetly sad and tediously resigned. She recites the stats on death and morbidity that we'll face tomorrow during administration of the anesthesia. The entourage smiles blissfully. "You're scheduled for another angiogram this morning. You've been told what that is, and you've already had one, but I'll tell you again. We go up from above the femoral artery to your brain, this time with radioactive dye. We'll give you a local anesthetic for this procedure, and it probably won't hurt you, but I have to tell you, you could die from this procedure. We've had people die during angiogram."

"What about morbidity?" I ask.

Dr. Theresa Smythe turns slowly my way and just as slowly nods, not in confirmation of morbidity but in sizing me up. "Yes, you could sustain morbidity in angiogram as well. But we can't be certain if the angiogram procedure would establish a cause and effect on the morbidity without . . ." She pauses, stopping short to keep from stepping in it.

"Without an autopsy? You know we're really sick of this shit."

"Of course you are. Have a nice day." They march out with most of the blissful entourage showing dents in their idiotic smiles. Nurse Nimmins shakes her head.

"All these young folk," I say, "calling themselves doctor. I'm not only unimpressed. I'm offended. These kids are way too full of themselves to be effective in the clutch or to know when to back down in the clutch. Whatever happened to humility and experience?"

"Your surgeon is that. Lawrence is the best. That's where it counts. You have to understand, this is a training hospital. That's why we have so many students. You're right. But they don't get next to the real procedures unless they're very good."

"I'm going to take a nap now," Rachel says, gently closing her eyes. My skin tightens. I look at Nurse Nimmins, who looks at the monitors and then at me with a nod. It's only a nap.

She whispers, "I'll be back." I ask how we can staunch the traffic. She nods and leaves, and the curtain remains undisturbed. I nod off as well but awaken every few minutes. Rachel sleeps so peacefully. I tense in the moments it takes to ascertain her breathing. In a while we both sleep. In another while the curtain opens again for Dr. Hsu, who tells us in her labored way that we will need speet patorogy after suhgely. This is nolmar, she says. We agree to everything, and she leaves, holding the curtain open for Sue, who has waited in the wings. I must tend to the dogs, take them for a pee and then take them home, back to the other side of Puget Sound.

"The dogs?" Rachel asks. "Where are they?"

I rehash the events of last night for her and assure her the dogs are fine. But I must go, if Sue can stay. The round trip will take me four hours. I'll make some calls on the way, to see if I can line up a house sitter. If I can't, well, we'll see.

An hour later I'm on the ferry with the dogs. I phone the ICU and get patched through. Rachel is gone. "What!" Gone to get her second angiogram.

Sue left soon after because, "There's nothing really you can do." Rachel will be back up in ICU in two more hours, or three.

I think only of logistics; otherwise I drift to what-ifs and the system clogs. I don't have Pamela's number but I know she works at the pizza place near the house. She's in, but she's already house sitting, but she knows three other women who might be available. If not, don't worry. She can come by morning and evening to feed the dogs and cats. I can't help the angst of imagining Dino and Molly in the cold and rain, outside all night. Another casualty could overload the system.

I arrive home to find the gate on the ground. It was broken last week by the mail carrier who tried to open it with her Jeep. Now it's fallen off the hinges, and though I can wrestle it back into place, it will need metal sleeves perpendicular to the through-bolts to keep the hinge pins vertically secure. I can cut the sleeves from ¾" pipe, available up the road only twenty miles at Home Improvement World.

I cannot doubt the wisdom of this errand nor challenge the tedium, nor can I hesitate. The gate serves no greater purpose than to keep the dogs alive, so I go, too easily imagining the impact of a death trifecta. No, first I stop and let the dogs pee and put them inside, but they cry and bark and whine, so I let them back out and into the car because dread and chaos is theirs to share along with the boredom of days on end, indoors. Now we go. They and the car whine for attention.

They want to go in with me but I tell them no. And stay. You stay. I stop at the espresso stand out front for a coffee, my first in two days. Or is it three? Or was that only yesterday? Never mind; I'll make this quick.

But once down aisle 23, I'm told that plumbing fixtures are on aisle 72, which is a fur piece in any country but could require navigational charts and a compass at Home Improvement World. Aisle 72 is not where it should be but way back to the southeast, from where I just came. Or did I enter there, to the northwest? I finally find a friendly clerk and get rerouted to conduit, which is what I needed all along, which is not aisle 72 but is back by the nursery, where aisle 111 will eventually be, once our expansion is complete, and homeowners can improve even more.

This is not the time to draw unsettling parallels between a medical industry outrunning its headlights and a building supply store with matching chaos and overload. I think I'm tolerating things reasonably well, considering the barrage of this place. Traffic jam and franchise foods clog the perimeters, inside and out. You can stop for a snack on your way to aisle after aisle of stuff in bulk. My wife is in a bunker with optic fibers running from her femoral artery through her heart to her left temporal lobe. The mail carrier triggered this—but not really. The mail carrier only facilitated a propitious timing, in which Rachel and I could slide down the rabbit hole to a place of . . . healing? I feel helpless and resentful but wonder what anger will accomplish. And what sense does it make anyway?

Yet I turn a corner to see a three hundred pound woman in a dress, ogling a whirlpool bath that she would fit into about as neatly as a hippo in a salad bowl. I don't begrudge her fantasy, but I see her as microcosm of our culture. She stares longingly at the whirlpool bath, gently plucking three sausage snack samples from the nearby server. The fancy tub is molded with lion's feet in the corners and sits three steps up on a display covered in fake marble to look like a Roman bath.

Did the Romans have snack samples at the ends of the aisles?

I think the world and my wife are dying, and that I may survive to a void—not a lovely void but a clutter of humanity short on hope or beauty. Maybe nature is bent on displacing bad thoughts. My first coffee since the crisis quickly swells my bladder. My eyes feel yellow. I have to piss like two cows on the same rock. I have to piss like a hydrant. I have to piss now.

And there is the toilet display. I pick a very fancy model in Forest Pine Mint, meaning green. Forest Pine Mint? Who is calling whom irrational? I think reality is changing its nature and I'm failing to adapt. Or am I? I drop my fly for a whiz. Looking natural keeps unwanted attention at a minimum. So I turn my back on the passing parade in its ebb and flow and look up, like I'm reading the sports page that is often tacked up over the urinals in some of your better bars and bistros.

Like all toilets in the display, this Forest Mint Pine model is unplumbed and will soon lead to another flow, call it Lemon Sunrise, or Double Tall Latte Piss. I can hear a few gawkers whispering gruffly, just as I image athletes hear isolated voices in the roar of the crowd— "Look at that man!" They sound rote and predictable part of the Home Improvement World without end. I doubt that my particular drummer is keeping a better beat and know I should stop, but pissing on the floor seems perfectly responsive to the mistreatment and neglect coming our way. The cats would have pissed in my shoes or dropped a load on the floor to prove a similar point. I feel felinely aligned if not justified; so bladder muscles get the OK from HQ, and even as I regret what we've come to, I ease on, because I'm more disgusted than most.

But a hand grasps my arm—gently against precision aim. It's connected to a white sleeve and on up to an orange vest and smiling old guy, who says, "Come on. We have one that works much better right over here." I feel compromised yet again, but he's so straightforward and simply communicative that I follow him mere paces to the men's room, where a solid whiz lets me rejoin the reasonable world.

The Home Improvement man waits at the door and tells me to have a great rest-of-your-day, as if whackos and wingnuts cuing up to display toilets are just another Tuesday around here. I nod in feeble assurance and tell him that I feel greatly relieved. "You guys promote full service so effectively that I believed it, and it's true." I head out feeling Home Improvement satisfaction as only a two-minute piss can provide.

I feel better about the rough treatment by a rigid society and would go back to tell him how his good deed helped my outlook. He watches, maybe looking out for a compulsive #2, and I realize as well that society is neither merciful nor repugnant but practical, sometimes to a fault. Me too. Fuck it. I exit south-southeast.

On aisle 61 I miraculously find ¾" pipe in four-foot lengths, which suggests spiritual guidance in a benignly indifferent world. The pipe is a solution to what ails us for now.

Four more friendly clerks in orange vests come around the far corner off aisle 17, which abuts aisle 37—go figure—adjacent to rough plumbing. They look intent, so I veer south, feeling like a dead-to-rights perp cruising conspicuously slowly in a White Bronco. At Customer Service a woman glances up, so I raise the pipe and put two twenties on the counter. "I don't have time for this." Her friendly smile is on the verge of advising a nice day, but she senses something amiss. In ten more paces I'm out.

Walking briskly to the car, I hear a voice in the distance, "Hey!" I can't be sure it's aimed at me and besides, hay is for horses. I learned that in third grade. I close the door in a flush of excitement—an odd blend of victory and guilt, like I've done something wrong and got away with it.

Molly and Dino are very happy that I've returned in a few minutes instead of seven hours. They whine and wag their tails and want to know if I brought them any biscuits. I promise them biscuits and a tad more anarchy at home as I gaze at them in another realization that anarchy has devolved to confusion. Where is my representative who'll take over in this time of dementia? Molly and Dino don't like such reflection, so they whine and lick and whine some more, taking over in their way.

The car fits right in, bonging higher decibels, flashing on the dash now as well as on the handy console data panel, insisting that I get professional help or face the reaper. I love ignoring it.

We speed home, and in another hour the gate is back up. It will make do for another week. In the meantime, Sandy left a message that yes, she's available. I call back, and she comes over. We review the drill, and in minutes I'm back on board the ferry for the ride across Puget Sound, quickly falling asleep.

My nap is deep but brief. In only minutes it's another rugged waking, another bonging and flashing in the traffic weave, back to Intensive Care. Rachel looks resentful, angry and pained. "Do you know what they did to me?"

"I do. I would give anything to have them do it to me instead."

"Easy for you to say."

"Yes, well. Tell me what you want me to do. I'll do it." She wants me to take her home. I feel like a politician, assuring her the home front is secure, the house sitter in place. She says again she's not sure she wants to do this.

I'm spared further dialogue by the curtain opening on Goldfarb again. "Hello. Is this a good time?" Rachel closes her eyes. I can't believe his gall. He makes pissing on the floor seem like child's play. He wants to assure us that he's reviewed our very special needs with the team, and all parties involved agree that two signatures on the consent form will serve everyone's best interest. I tell him that we're resting now. It's not a good time. We're trying to conduct a nap here. If he could give us, say, a week and a half?

"He's not writing anything," Rachel says.

"We want this to be a family involvement. That way you won't be alone."

"I'm not having surgery," she says.

"Not having surgery? You must."

She shakes her head. "That's not what they said at the store."

Goldfarb loves the volley with an apparent handicap on the other side of the net. "You're not fluent!" he trumpets. "You must have surgery. And you both must sign."

"Dr. Goldfarb. She's fluent. She's not lucid. Never has been. You want lucid; you talk to me. But not now. Now we really must invite you to leave." Goldfarb is troubled. "I'm afraid we'll have to insist."

Goldfarb doesn't need the hostility, and neither do I. Fortunately, into the tension steps the neurosurgeon. "Do we have the consent?" he asks. "What's the delay?" He looks at me. "Do you want to proceed or not? We're very busy."

I take the consent form from Goldfarb. "We want to proceed. Rachel, sign this please."

"What does it say?"

"It says you're fully informed on the possibility of mortality and morbidity, and you won't sue."

"Am I?"

I smile at her. "Yes. You am."

She signs. I address the surgeon. "We've had a meeting of the minds for a while now, Doctor Lawrence. Goldfarb here seems hell bent on a pissing contest, but if it's all the same to you, we're feeling the need for some peace and quiet while we wait for surgery."

The neurosurgeon takes the consent with a nod. I have not signed. "Best we get on with it," he says.

"I agree."

Goldfarb leaves. The neurosurgeon has the angiogram negative with him for review with us. This is not customary, but I learn that in my absence Rachel has threatened to leave again if she can't see the negative and see her name on it and have it explained by the man who proposes to penetrate her skull and probe her brain. I've always known that her social skills outpace my own, and I'm frankly relieved that she's sharing the burden here.

Dr. Lawrence explains, pointing out the primary vessels and bifurcations. The aneurysm dangles like a bloated grub, obviously out of synch in nature's arabesque of vessels in a gossamer-like web that feeds the brain. We are further instructed on the insight gained by angiogram, which is a clear view of the vessel network. The view of the veins is unencumbered by the clot, thanks to the angiogram. We are told the aneurysm is bigger than anticipated; these things are rated technically as small, moderate, large and huge. This one is huge, a veritable mystery of nature, to stretch so far and not burst but only leak. It's nine millimeters long, five millimeters wide.

It's been there for years, possibly since birth. I want to tell Dr. Lawrence that the long-term nature of the thing was my initial hunch, contrary to that of young Dr. Michael, but I stay mum. "You see how the aneurysm dangles forward and slightly in? That means it bled into the space around the brain. If it dangled forty degrees the other way, it would have bled into the brain, causing instant death."

"How much of my head will you cut off?"

He looks dismayed. "She means hair."

He smiles. "I'll do my best. I promise. I'll cut as little as possible. But we must cut some."

"Can I pull it over to the other side and hold it with a beret. Or tie it with a rubber band?"

"No berets or rubber bands in the OR. You'll have to trust me."

"Show me again where you'll cut me."

Again he drags his finger from behind the part in her hair, around and down. "About nine inches," he says. But he sees the downward spiral in this line of questioning, so he gives us good news; the aneurysm, though large, appears to be a single weak spot in the cell wall and not a cluster. A compromised bifurcation often appears with smaller bubbles off the vessel wall with a bleeding aneurysm. When these occur, they must also be fixed as long as the brain is exposed, which adds complexity and several more paragraphs of disclosure on the statistical history of mortality and morbidity during surgery. We have been spared the smaller bubbles, however.

"You mean they can be like rhoids?"

"Like what?"

"Hemorrhoids. You know how they want to bunch up on you once they get started?"

"Not exactly. But if that helps you, then yes."

Why not like rhoids? I think it's exactly like rhoids. Never mind. We're signed off and won't be disturbed between now and then. Lawrence of Neurology turns away with a smile over his shoulder. "You can eat tonight. Not tomorrow. Not too spicy. You're on the dietitian's rounds for dinner. They'll be by in a little while."

7

---◆◆◆---

The Gift of the Ages

It's not for nothing that hospitals are known for bad food. Still, you hope it's only a joke, but then you know it's not when the dietitian arrives with the evening shmush. She's a roly-poly, jolly lass who appears to do the tasting and spend her days off at FoodCo buying in bulk. She delivers this meal in person to introduce herself. Dinner is two slices of white bread smashed under a fillet of sole, meaning shoe sole dba "prime rib." The assemblage is drowned in cream gravy with a lightly congealed skin.

I laugh. I know I shouldn't, but it's a blessing, the laughter. The sight, scent and sound of it ("Oh, God . . .") make this a wonder to behold. Rachel minds her manners but tells the dietitian, "I don't eat meat."

"Aw-hall right then. That's why I'm here, to make sure everything is just how you like it. Vegetarian. Okay. Do you eat dairy products?"

"Yes. And fish and chicken are all right."

"Okey dokey. I'll take care of that." The dietician takes her leave, leaving us to hunt or gather dinner for ourselves. Maybe it's a good night for a continuing fast. Or maybe Rachel will get hungry enough to eat what she's been served.

I check the rest of dinner, which is green gelatin, coffee and four slabs of butter. "And no coffee," I yell. "And low fat!" Too late. The dietitian is gone to see that tomorrow turns out better.

"I haven't eaten in three days," Rachel says. I agree, though it's really only two days. What does she want? Nothing is what she wants. But that's not such a good idea.

Why not?

Well, because it's good to have something to eat before they slice your melon open. This I don't say, because the curtain opens again on a cheery face and a happy voice along with bright eyes and good posture. I hope for the best but I brace for goo goo morbidity talk or more extraneous blather.

"Hel-lo. I'm Leah, your new nurse. I only have one other patient tonight, but he might need me fairly regular. He's a little guy, banged his head pretty badly."

"Still no vacancy in neurology ICU?"

"No. We bring the kids here anyway, no matter what their injury. Did you get dinner?"

"Well. Yes and no," I say. Leah understands; she saw it. I ask where is good for take out, nearby. She says the Thai place a mile down is good. Rachel likes the idea, but wants it simple, maybe some noodles, maybe some . . . pineapple. No, not pineapple, some . . . What do you call it?

Tofu?

Yes, tofu. Not too spicy. Leah assures us this place has good tofu. She feels like a lucky draw; she's so normal, yet I wonder why she would choose a life of days and nights in this place.

It's dark outside, wet and windy, and the medivac helicopter is grinding to earth again from somewhere in five states, delivering another trauma victim. I lean into the slanting rain and cinders and feel the little stings bouncing off the numbness of days and nights of no sleep and no beer.

I find the Thai place and order thirty bucks worth of this and that and a beer, right now if you don't mind. The Thai fellow at the cash register watches me inhale the beer. I wonder if my color improves as I return marginally to where I once belonged. He shags another without being asked, pops the top and says, "Slow down. Plenty time." I obey, drinking the second one. It gives me goose bumps, perhaps relieving a minor withdrawal or filling a fundamental need or taking the edge off or taking whatever form fulfillment needs to take. It tastes like a consolation, like a gift from nature. I finish when the groceries arrive, and the man says, "You like one more?"

"Well, to tell you the truth I think I might."

He shags a brown bag and puts the beer inside. "Must not open for you to take out."

"I understand." I've already paid, but when I go to pay for this one, he pops the top and waves me off. I am taken by small kindness in my time of need. Sure, I gave him thirty bucks for some noodles and tofu and a half-dozen shrimp, but still. I walk back to the car through teeming throngs of alternate-sexual-preference kids with rings, pins, staples, and cotter keys piercing their faces. I feel their pain and wonder if mine shows.

I feel better on my return, though it's after eight. Visiting hours are over, so I must walk in the wind and rain around the complex to the night entrance, where security is tighter than at the UN. I am interrogated, scanned, frisked and finally approved.

Up in the ICU Rachel is napping but opens her eyes and says, "I can smell it." She opens a box ravenously, eats four bites then lays back and sighs.

"That's it?"

"I'm full. I haven't eaten in days."

I haven't either. Nor am I the beneficiary of several gallons of electrolytes through four IV tubes. I eat. But I too fill quickly. And I tire. I watch her drift off, and I ease on back in the chair, apparently undetected on the ICU. We sleep.

I awaken in the night in a pleasant drift with no coordinates; with no intersect on the space/time continuum. I am nobody on an extended visit to nowhere. Momentarily lost and free-floating, I'm quickly found. Compression wakens me to the density of earthly mass closing in. Flashing lights, beeps and the wail of humans remind me of vital function run amok.

We are in a hospital, Intensive Care. My neck is so stiff I must sit up slowly. I have to whiz so badly I must slowly stand. I wish for a mint julep raspberry daiquiri toilet display in the hall, and I laugh. But I stop, because I really have to whiz, and because I must keep my suburban adventure to myself or get yelled at. This I know, ducking behind the curtain to the commode. Nurse Leah is changing occluded quart bottles, meaning empty, when I emerge, refreshed. "You were sleeping pretty hard," she says. "You guys have been up a few days, huh?"

I nod. "I'm breaking the rules, being here, aren't I?"

"Nah. You can leave whenever you're ready. It doesn't matter. I think you'll be better off tomorrow if you can get some sleep though." I love her; her language and demeanor are so reasonable and understanding. Or maybe she simply knows how to handle a customer like me. Either way is okay.

From deep in her covers, Rachel asks, "Am I still on for eleven?"

"Yes, you are. But time doesn't mean anything here. Everyone gets bumped. But I know they'll get you in there at some point tomorrow."

"How do you know?" I ask.

With a tight-lipped smile she says, "You're at sixty hours."

"You mean . . ."

She nods. "Since the bleed. That's very important." She touches me. "Get some rest. I'll take good care of your sweetie."

"They won't let me wash my head when it's done, will they?" Rachel is up from the covers now, perhaps sensing the goal line.

"No. But I'll tell you what; we'll wash it in the morning. Okay?"

"You'll help me?"

"You bet I will."

Rachel rolls over and softly says, "They want to cut it off."

Leah bends beside her and says, "I know how you feel. I know what it's like for you two. They don't know what to make of you."

"You do?"

"Yes. Maybe not exactly how you feel. But I was in here last year for three weeks. If the staff stayed here like I did and like you are, they'd understand."

"What was wrong with you?"

"Collapsed lung. They don't know why. I'm fine now. Believe me, you're doing the right thing. I've never heard of anything for what you have besides surgery."

"You're familiar with alternative remedies?"

Leah blushes. "Not like you are. I wish I knew more. I'm learning. I can tell you though; they do this procedure every day, sometimes two or three a day. They're really good, and your surgeon is the best. He's so grounded. They're all assholes, you know. Not him."

I think the hospital should can the shrink and hire Leah; in two minutes flat she's brought us over, calmed us and helped us accept what we must.

"Lawrence has no sense of humor," I note.

"You really don't need that in a surgeon. Believe me, he won't leave anything disfigured. In six months you won't even see it."

"Six months?" Rachel says. "It'll take ten years to grow back."

"No, it won't. I've seen it. You'll see. I have to go check my little guy. You two get some rest."

"I . . ." Rachel begins, then checks herself, then she concedes, "I have a headache."

It's another four. Leah records it plus the Tylenol.

We wait, as if for the headache to depart. Rachel is nodding off now, so I bend near for a sweet goodnight. I am saddened yet again by her fear of hair loss. I tell her to rest easy, I'm turning in but I'll be back first thing. In the meantime I'm only minutes away. She insists that I take my time tomorrow. In fact I should plan to go out and do something else. I should have some fun.

"You mean like cruise a few bars and go shopping?"

"Yeah. Get out of here. I would."

"Well. I might. Later. But right now this is what I'm doing. So if you don't mind, I'll see you in the morning."

"I don't mind. I just . . . I don't want to . . ."

"No. I don't either. But here we are."

She sits halfway up. "I don't want to do this."

"I know. I don't either. Let's take tonight off and review it in the morning." To my surprise she eases back down, in agreement, I hope.

In ten minutes I'm ten blocks away in my office on the ninth floor watching the city lights blink profusely, hearing the wind howl outside. I drink a soda to quell the nausea and a brandy to numb the pain. Tomorrow is only a handful of hours away, and I seek a different feeling, call it understanding or acceptance or something that might make sense, something that will let me know why this is happening. I can't find it, can't make contact with the reality surrounding us, yet I sense a continuing, other presence.

I call my brother in St. Louis to tell him the news. He asks if he should fly out. I ask why. To help, he says. I'll let him know, I say. If she dies or suffers a stroke in surgery, then yes, I'll need help.

But we're cut off. I call back, and the line is dead.

I call his cell phone, and he asks what the hell was that. What was what? He says his phone jacks popped like firecrackers and blew sparks out of the wall, and now he thinks his regular phone is fried. He wants me to call tomorrow. I promise to do so.

A spirit is here, around me and in me. It taunts me, perhaps in response to my invitation, one on one. It howls at the gates. I offered a tussle. Now it cackles, ready to feed. Call me old fashioned, but I recognize the ethereal world apart, in which luck takes a header or a lift, depending on variables. My old Aikido teacher once said the dark ones made trouble for his ninety-five year old mother, until he made them go away. What did he do? He had no choice in the matter; he had to get rid of them. How did he do it? He yelled at them.

So for the second time in a long, long day I challenge the laws of modern society in abeyance to the laws of a different nature. I open the slider and step into the breeze. My skin tingles in the clammy air—forty-two degrees and windy. I feel affirmed of the shadowy presence, and I erupt: "Get out! Out and awaaaaay! Go! Go! Go away!" I follow quickly with the sentiment that is most felt inside. "Eeeyyyiiiaaaahhh! Ahhh! Ahhhh! Ahhhh! Go away from here! Go away! Eeeeyiaaa!"

A few lights go on across the way. I'm shaking as I yell at the top of my lungs to get out, get away from here and go away. Go back to where you belong!

I want to feel that something is changed, but I cannot.

I go back inside and lie down. I drift on a new understanding of life and death these few thousand years it's been around. I understand something other than what I want to understand. I think that among the gifts of the ages is the unspoken but widely practiced rule that old people don't remind the young ones too often of the end and how it slams into you not all that long after you were only just nineteen, and all the days merge into one.

And all the days of our lives are but a single breath. They pass at the end of a single day. I remember that part from the Yiskor service for the dead on Yom Kippur. I considered it an exaggeration for years—how can a life filled with proper wine, song, adventure and laughter pass so casually and briefly at the end? Yet here we are, facing the end.

Oh, I'll most likely survive tomorrow and a few years besides with minimal mortality and morbidity. But what about my friend, my mate, my alter ego and confidant? Is she not a part of me? She is, and I feel so worthless in my efforts.

Only on Yom Kippur do the Jews let the truth be known to the young. Even reminded annually I never took it to heart. After all, Yom Kippur is a consciously solemn time in which gravity itself is the point. The truth of the quickness of the end is dispensed like a harsh medicine and is diluted by the pomp and certain knowing that soon we will eat. What else can a religion do, bring you down? Well, it does bring you down, but only in a deliberate way that is blessedly brief with an uplift at the end. This, on the other hand, remains unknown.

I understand now; you can't prepare for the end, you can only strive for calmness and repose. You might keep your mind clear. Then you go. Calmness is what I seek, and clarity, yet I cry again at the loss of the fun we should have had.

But I'm pressing the issue, accepting the worst, which indicates the continuing presence of you-know-who. I set aside these thoughts of mortality and morbidity, which isn't easily done without something to take their place. So I close my eyes and mount up, keeping time now with a different beast that pounds poetry beneath me. Rachel is on back, where she's ridden thousands of miles, and through the night we cruise the countryside under the stars, sweeping the vast plateau.

I'm neither sentimental nor optimistic, yet the dawn comes with certain knowing that things are changed. I open my eyes and feel the change. I rise like a tin man after a spring rain and shuffle to the slider. It opens on a continuing chill breeze and confirmation that the dark spirit is gone. I cannot explain what I know, but I hurriedly shower, dress and get to the hospital to share the news.

Three people inside the curtain are busy. One is our nurse. Another is emptying the trash and sweeping and another is writing in a notebook. Our new nurse came on at the shift change and is a sobering, perfunctory presence in contrast to Nurse Leah, who stayed twenty minutes past shift change to keep her promise and assist with a hair wash.

Rachel was in better spirits then but already suffers the new nurse. As he changes electrolyte bottles, she enumerates his faults. He has a dour outlook and is rough with her IV connections. He tangles the sheets and mumbles complaints. She told him to go away and don't come back. He said he'd be out of this place in three more days, and he only wanted to get through them. She told him he was awful, and if he had to scowl all the time he shouldn't be around people who need help, who don't need a sourpuss so full of himself he can't see farther than his own petty needs.

Then he smiled and was nice, but it was too late; she doesn't like him and doesn't want him around. She fears this bitter fellow for his discouraging essence, which can envelope the weak and lamenting. I ask him what time his shift ends. He says eleven. I tell him great, we'll share the shift. He reads me easily and minds his manners.

Then again, a sourpuss on the ward may be a healthy distraction to the gang valve pumping the four leads in her jugular. A three-inch slice in her neck facilitated insertion, and a few sutures hold things snug so the hardware won't frag loose on an emotional outburst. The package is wrapped in transparent tape. Rachel takes the beating, whining infrequently over what would make a strong man weak. But her internal struggle reaches new levels. As her eyes grow heavy with sad resignation, she achieves what the shrink would call acceptance, which he apparently thinks is good. To me, she seems on the verge of giving up.

"I don't want to do this," she says.

"I know you don't. I don't either."

"Take me home."

"You know I will."

"Now. Take me now."

"I can't now. But I will. You know I will."

"I don't care if . . . You know . . . I just don't want to . . . die here." Her facial muscles turn down like when she was a baby and couldn't control them and expressed herself the only way she could, without words, because the words wouldn't come out right, and besides, nobody was listening. Down to a frown she makes me want to change things, anything to relieve the load. Tears flow into heavy sobs now.

She wrestles the dark spirit herself. Pain tightens my chest and throat, and I blurt the only words available to halt our downward spiral. "I peed on the floor at Home Improvement World."

"You what?" She wipes her eyes, checks the anguish and moves quickly to a brow beating.

"Yes. They got me so . . . irritated, you wouldn't believe it."

"So you pissed on the floor?"

"Yes," I laugh now with a few tears of my own. "It sounds much worse when you say it like that."

"Like what?"

"Like, you know, I pissed on the floor."

"That's what you said."

"It wasn't that bad."

"You're sick."

"I don't think I'm sick." I want to explain the short circuit in my perception of society, but the next realization is that short circuitry and not-knowing the why or wherefore of a thing can be part of a greater process. I want to recant—to beg off my claim and state the truth of pissing on the floor, but the idea is a far greater gift than the act could ever have been. I feel alienated as ever from the world of better living and fat women fantasizing soaking tubs and unplumbed toilets that beckon me for a piss. Yet I come home to the profound truth that events are nothing up next to the effect of a good story. So I offer pitiful affirmation of a numbing disconnection. "I really had to piss."

"That's terrible!" she says.

"I know." I hang my head. "Terrible. But practical. I wanted to take a dump but held back. Maybe I'm not hopeless."

She scans for sick humor and may sense a bit, but I do share her concern. Goldfarb entering again spares us further scrutiny. I've made an impression on him too; his smile is tight, and he offers no apology. "I'm only putting this page in the chart. Thank you." He slips his page in quietly and leaves.

Rachel is calmer now. She regrets my behavior, telling me it was wrong and she's disappointed. I agree that it was wrong and that disappointment was a factor for me too. "Yes, disappointed, but it was a small rebellion, and it did dilute my bigger disappointment. It was a distraction. I was acting out, killing the rules that drive me crazy."

"You didn't have to go crazy or make pee pee on the floor." She is curt and final.

"You know I don't like much in life."

"I know. It's too bad."

"Yes, it is, but I'm disgusted."

"You don't exactly help the situation."

"I know. But I can't help it. I do like some things—a few cats, some dogs, my motorcycle, you—I love those things. I think I love them too much because I have so few places to put my love, so things stack up on me more than the average bear. So it's tough. This is the toughest yet."

She takes my hand. She kisses it. "I'm only fourth on the list?"

"It's a strong fourth."

She smiles, musing on springtime, on the first sunny day in weeks, and look at where she is. I tell her it's not sunny; that's only glare. She points to a break in the clouds and asks what flowers are blooming in the garden. I forgot to notice, but the tulips should be showing, or at least the tulip buds. She picks up her knitting and knits. I open a book and stare off. We share this repose for a few hours until eleven-thirty, when the shift changes and the new nurse comes in.

She says everything is on schedule. I tell her we were scheduled for eleven, and it's eleven-thirty. She says scheduling here means only that things occur in sequence, but the sequence can change, and a changed sequence changes timing, because urgent traumas arrive non-stop. Sequence is not bound to a clock. So it's good that we have some knitting and reading material. So we knit and nap till one, then two, then three. Rachel wants me to go.

"Go where?"

"Out somewhere. Have some fun."

"What's with you and fun?"

She points out that this is such a drag.

"Yeah, well, life has its draggy days. Leave me alone, will you?"

And with a sweep of the curtain, in comes the nurse to tell us it's show time.

Yes, I can come along. We're only going now to pre-op, which will take an hour or so with general prep and the sedative administered prior to anesthesia. I'm apprehensive in general terms, like a fighter before a big one, and it's not even on me. I succeed in hiding my fear, for my mate's face shows the elusive calmness that the most diligent monks take years to achieve. She's ready in all ways. I suspect this readiness has been there for years, is possibly genetic. The new nurse gathers loose ends, the books, pamphlets, knitting, make-up, berets and rubber bands. We're not checking out, just moving on. The nurse stacks things near the chart, which I pick up and open. "Not supposed to do that," she says.

I smile. "Who is this information about?" I ask.

She smiles back. Enough said. I turn to the last page, the one recently inserted by Goldfarb. It reads:

. . . Both she and husband discuss an 'AMA philosophy' which feels overwhelming, impersonal and offensive.

Now patient feels she has had conflicting information from other staff and is worried.

PATIENT IS PARANOID.

I back up a few pages and find the entry written by Lawrence of Neurology:

Of note, we have discussed the nature of this operation (L. crani for aneurysm clipping) alternative treatments, and the benefits + risks (including, but not limited to infection, bleeding, and death) of surgery with the pt. + her husband + they have signed consent to proceed.

Three signatures follow: Rachel's, the neurosurgeon's and Goldfarb's. Another chart with one-word classifications sits near the computer. Another word is hand-written in all caps: PARANOID. How's that for objective response?

In mere moments we're packed and ready, but the nurse tells us we must wait for an escort from the OR. I don't say that we know where it is, because the staff is weary of us. And I don't mind waiting a bit. On her way out the nurse turns the overhead TV on, so the most addictive drug known can sedate us for this brief interlude.

The TV brightens on an Executive Chef from the Ritz Carlton on (Ah . . .) Maui! The chef is a four hundred pounder with small liver spots but enormous panache. He packs a plucked squab from the hind opening with his famous garlic ginger plum sauce, which is thick as hot fudge. The bird's head and feet are still on, perhaps for culinary drama to quell kitchen ennui. The feet are bound at the ankles so the bird can dangle from a bamboo skewer, and into the hot box it goes for an hour at 350°. The big chef has failing teeth but can hardly suppress a famous grin for the famous verdict: *Mmm . . . Scrumptious!*

The bird seems familiar, plucked and poked to the point of desecration, then hastily prepped for a slow bake at 350° by a short-order crew dedicated to excellence. We cut to an hour later and the result: an exotic entrée with empty eye sockets stretched ankles and pointed toes curled and golden crispy.

Alas, our guide is here. He's very fat and has bad teeth—not really; I made that up, though I want to stop time, so heartily do I fear its lapse. We move toward the exit in orderly fashion. Competing images suggest the unwelcome presence again among us—our route feels like the walk from death row to the little room of finality, or a bridal party heading from the anteroom to the great hall of reverence. I dispense with both; the images are all in me, dark and otherwise. I wait for the orderlies and nurses to go first, and I take inventory. Everything seems in order, except for the felt-pen board hanging between the windows, where I write: *Just because you're paranoid doesn't mean they don't want to cut you up.* I hurry to catch up.

We descend.

Pre-op feels tense, beginning with the head woman whose name could be Dirk, who has the hair and face and aggressive demeanor of a professional wrestler. She pegs me and says, "You'll have to leave now. We can't have family in here."

"Yes. I understand." But I don't; it's not a sterile environment, and I sense a man problem between us.

"Now."

I step near and advise, "Back off."

She moves around me with a grunt. Nearby is a jovial scene, all the nurses, docs and orderlies scrubbing and joking, locking eyes or rubbing thighs or touching elsewhere, as seen on TV. What else can they do, despair?

Next.

All prepped for surgery, a patient rolls up on a gurney, pop-eyed and gape-mouthed as a sports fan at the playoffs. *This* patient is unconscious, but his eyes are open. *This* is why we can't have family in here. The patient is intubated, with a plastic tube down his throat to avoid aspiration, or puking, which is fatal under anesthesia. This patient is left in front of us while his advance guides interface with his team. Rachel stares at him, then at me.

I move into the crowd swarming my mate. They prep for incisions, stick new lines into her legs, add a couple to the gang valve in her neck, then pull her hair aside and glop the antiseptic. They roll her to one side and hike her jammies. Goose bumps rise on her ass, and she trembles, but a monotone voice issues assurance that this exposure is necessary for the spinal taps. We'll have two, to draw just a liiitle bit of spinal fluid, hardly a pint off the top to reduce cranial pressure, just in case, you know.

They don't stop but move quick and efficient as piranha on a piglet—stop that! I regret this imagery too and try to calm the waters, though pre-op pares emotions to the bone. A single tear wells in Rachel's eye, and she says, "There's more dog food in the basement and cat food across from the counter—"

"Sh . . ." I bend near and whisper, "Call on me. I'm with you. All my heart and all my soul."

She smiles. "Why don't you talk to me like that all the time?" Even on the cutting board she bats her eyes and complains of insufficient romance.

I shrug. "You know me. I speak off the top, and this feeling is coming right now."

"I love you very much," she says.

"You'd be a fool not to," I reply. "And I love you. I always will." We move together for a kiss, a light blending of lips and pulse in love with electricity arcing. I often think of our first kiss and think of it now, but then, like life, it seems so quickly gone.

Then again it's not, even when it is.

Our eyes lock as a haze sweeps over and leads me out through the swinging doors. I wipe my eyes, and see that it's Nurse Nimmins navigating for me. She walks me to the OR dispatch and introduces Anne, who just came on for the next eight hours. I'm instructed to ask for Anne when I call for updates and status. Anne doesn't stop talking on her headset but smiles and nods assuredly. I write *Anne* on piece of paper and pocket it.

I'm walked to the waiting room at Two West. "You should leave," Rebecca Nimmins says. "There is absolutely nothing you can do here, and you'll be in much better shape for her when she comes out of recovery, if you can get away from here and relax."

It's now four o'clock Friday afternoon. Rachel won't be out of surgery for six hours, then another hour or two in recovery. So we're looking at eleven-thirty or midnight.

"But I should be here," I say.

"You can't do anything here," she says.

I look away. She watches me. I look back. "What if she dies?" I ask. "I think I should be here."

Nurse Nimmins is a head taller than me. With a very sad look she says, "She's not going to die." I nod, hardly sanguine but receptive to the first affirmation from hospital staff since our arrival. I can't bank on kind words, but they allow the muscles to let go, to slump around the elusive belief that all will end well. I offer my hand in tentative farewell. Perhaps she sees my weakness and says, "I feel like I should hug you." I don't decline, so she steps up and wraps her arms around me, and against her gentle bosom I tremble.

8

The Angels Sing

Yay, though I walk through the Valley of the Shadow, I fear less than I did on the approach. Once into a thing you tend to process it more easily, beyond the angst. My doubts and concerns are nothing next to those of my mate. Whatever I stand to lose, she stands to lose more. Together we face the third potential: a life together but apart from life as we know it. In place of the carefree life, we may live with caregivers, attendants and nurses for years to come.

The team seems intent on processing the difficulty we presented. The effect of their effort is negative; our difficulty stems from their difficulty. Ignorance is not bliss, but obfuscation and condescension are ambient. Every inquiry made in the last three days was met with statistical disclosure. I suspect it's all they have—or all they're allowed. We don't share the need for legal precaution but remain keen on quality in life. We are skeptical of medical miracles. We were made to feel foolish for expecting a role in the process, an emergency process resulting from years of trial and error in a healthcare system dominated by the legal system, the insurance system, the drug industry and the medical complex as it defers to all of the above in its quest for maximum billings. We have suffered a loss of spirit as debilitating as our fear of life lost or impaired.

You can never know what your mate is thinking, yet I'd bet the farm that she agrees. We are noted as paranoid for lack of utter, blind faith in this place—for asking questions repeatedly, because we got no answers.

I never faulted Rachel's vanity. She's too selfless in other ways. So what if she's a classic beauty who feels good with her good looks, who has fun with what has come her way? Can I call this a character defect in a woman who would pull to the grassy center divider of an interstate highway to rescue a duck and six ducklings? Do I label her self-absorbed after seeing her make a bed in the bathtub so a three-legged bitch could recover from the amputation? "This dog is only six," she said, "and besides, she wants me to do this." And besides, all the kennels at the pound are full, and a three-legger would be going down.

It's the same way with a huge blue macaw accused of attacking hotel personnel on the lawn of the Grandiose Arms, or whatever silly name the place goes by—landed right there out of the clear blue sky and tried to bite the boys who only wanted to bag him. Could someone come down and, you know, subdue him or put him down or whatever it is that you do? Oh, yes, Rachel could go. With a smile on her face and love in her heart she marched past the boys and mid-managers up to the big bird and offered a forearm. Simon (the bird) looked down and off to one side. Then he stepped on up to the shoulder, where he rode for a year until Lily came along, another huge blue who'd plucked half her feathers from sheer frustration from living in solitary confinement but got sprung at last on an abuse charge. Simon and Lily became an item in Rachel's living room—Lily stopped plucking, and next thing you know, it's a nesting family in a plastic dog kennel fitted behind their cage. Three little baby macaws taking the bottle were far from home in the treetops of South America where they belonged, but they'd also arrived, equidistant from the misery their parents had suffered. Is this vanity?

So what if Rachel can't walk or dress or feed herself? So what if she lives in a wheel chair? Will she not remain the Queen of Hearts? Yes, she will, but I set these thoughts aside, for I feel the foul spirit seeking openings that open wider here.

The team prepared us for the very worst so we can't say we weren't warned. I think the spirits, dark and otherwise, go like luck, where they are most received. I think the team knows the numbers, and I sense a practiced and practical numbness among them, even those who freely show optimism. I'm sure the numbness is required by the job, and I'm not the first guy to whistle in the dark.

I stand on the street corner by the Emergency Room door. I bum a cigarette from a pedestrian and smoke it with the other bums.

I sit in my car in the parking lot with the engine running. It bongs, lights flashing for service, but I want the heater on.

I stare out my window on the ninth floor in downtown Seattle. Ships go out in search of the world and come back in.

I lie back on the sofa and stare at the ceiling. I watch my thoughts. An hour goes by and another.

I get up and light incense, nine sticks of it, three each for the three levels of the spirit recognized in Huna magic, the way of Aloha. I light four more sticks for the four seasons and four more for the winds and one more for Rachel. I stand in the smoke and pull it over me because I've seen Indians do this in the movies—real Indians, our Indians.

The phone rings and wrings my wits, shattering the trance like a hand grenade on my desk.

"Hello."

"Hey, man."

"Hey. I got a bad situation."

"I know. How is she?"

"In surgery."

"Keith told me. When did she go in?"

"Four."

"Can I come down?"

"Yeah. Why don't you."

"See you in a bit."

"Hey. Call before you come up. I might go on back down there."

"You can't do anything down there. Let's relax for a while."

"Fine. If I'm not here, I'll be down there. Two West."

He agrees but encourages me to hang around the office for another few hours, because it's so much more comfortable, and the waiting rooms are a drag, and you can't even smoke a joint there. He's my friend, Stuey Stuart, with whom I ride motorcycles, if not to live then at least to forget. Or maybe we ride to remember how it was when school was out and the world was ours.

I need a friend now for distraction, even as I fear his brand of distraction. But I want to drop the fear; what could be better to displace a focus on mortality and morbidity than the distraction Stuey usually offers? What else can you do in life but live? He brings casual confidence to the table, whether we face brain surgery or a pass on a twisty mountain road in torrential rain. We'll press on to a fire in the hearth. He's good for that. Still, he's worse than a wife when it comes to prepping for an outing. He could be two hours with his face and his hair, and I pace, waiting for the phone to ring again, hoping against the worst but ready for action if it comes. Then I head down.

I scan the office before leaving to double check what should be second nature, things like the lights, the oven, the refrigerator, because I'm forgetful now, absent-minded and severely distracted. The stove is off, and so are the lights—but wait. Rachel made the glass lampshades in the office, nouveau flower patterns in predominant blues with red and orange petals and green leaves. I go to the two by the reading chair she uses when she waits for me to finish my work. I turn them on and place my palms on the shades, feeling the space where her hands once worked, feeling the lingering neurons—feeling what people in Hawaii would call the energy. I take my leave and leave those lights on.

Of course this is human nature, the one based on hope and desire. We will die like the other animals do and join them in drinking what Socrates called the waters of forgetfulness. Then it won't matter. I knew this and accepted it long ago, yet I hope and desire.

Maybe it's the starvation diet and sleep deprivation of the last few days on top of the impact and rapid descent to mortality/morbidity potential. I'm leveled out now, the G-forces of ignition and liftoff more manageable, but that which surrounds me feels surreal. The walls don't breathe, nor do the floors tilt to a corner where I could roll down the drain. Yet I stand on the rim of a deep, dark hole. I pinch myself and it feels like a pinch. My senses seem in tact, yet I feel removed. I recall the times when death seemed near, only twice for me. The first close encounter was on acid, when a six-foot pepperoni pizza festering purple cheese chased me down the road.

The second was at sea, inescapable as the first with no alternative but to ride it out and remember Mother as the bulkheads cracked. Those moments never go away. Yet I think this current proximity takes a greater toll. The potential death is not my own, but I feel more stuck than before. Before, I could measure the difficulty and adjust, more or less. I could go for a walk or trim the rig or check the hatches or clean the bilge-pump filter again or smoke a joint or drink some wine to dull the edge. Now I want to move my mind off dead center, but I can't. I can't help her or me. I am helpless.

An elderly woman steps onto the elevator and stares at me. I don't know why, until I realize she is only staring back. Oh, and she's waiting for a response to her greeting. "How are you?" I tell her I'm fine so she can proceed with her thoughts on the weather.

I step out of the elevator into the garage and walk toward my car but stop halfway, alone, with these few cars and God. I listen and wonder why the world offers no more silence except in a parking garage four levels underground. "Okay," I ask. "What do you want?"

The question blurts out. "What do you want? Tell me what you want." I don't address a personal God. I hold humans and their personal needs and the God who exists to fulfill these things as the source of most trouble in the world. I am here in trouble on a personal level. Yet in the crux I won't give in, for it would be nothing but weakness. I have faith in what I know, so I seek strength through answers available in nature. That is, I beckon for guidance. It will come, if you let it. I stand still. It doesn't come, so I ask myself what I must do. And I weaken, finally promising to be "good" forever, if only . . .

I know that won't get it either; what is "good" to me would be damnable to the teeming refuse yearning to be free. I press on to the world outside, with its pavement and construction and unyielding demand for more. I vow on the way to renew my commitment to personal goodness, if only ...

Dusk on Friday is jammed with traffic, people hurrying to flee this congestion for its suburban counterpart. A dense sky moves slowly in all directions like traffic verging on critical mass. Light is a concept here. This is daytime in Seattle, mostly characterized by glare in shades of gray, dirty scud to gunmetal to thunderhead.

I creep slowly in the non-flow to a red light. Two lanes over on the bus a black woman meets my eyes. We look away and then down at a man between us in a late-model sedan with a sunroof, picking his nose. Digging upward for a stubborn woolly one, he finally hooks it, plays it light and draws it on out. He stares at it on his fingertip as the bus woman and I bunch our foreheads, and then he eats it—sucks it off his finger with relish. We gasp in unison. She looks at me again from two lanes over and shrieks *Oh, God!* And we laugh, moving apart because the light is green.

At the next light I see a silver-haired man in a silver suit and matching Porsche twiddle a mint from its silver wrapper and eat it. Maybe he had eggs for lunch, and now his breath smells like mint and sulfur. Or maybe he ate his secretary for lunch. Or his boyfriend. Or maybe he's sucking antacid tabs to dull the edge in his gut after a day of risking megabucks for more. Green again, and we're off. Every Joe Blow in town needs to ace a Porsche in first gear. Me too, until I slow and give him his due, staying calm, being good.

The waiting room in Two West is fifty by fifty with one door and no windows. Families wait here. It's a grief collective but with separate scripts, each group tuned uniquely to the vicissitudes of old age or car wreck or untimely disease or more exotic trauma. I take a seat at the deep end, seeking space and clean air. Two boys in their twenties sit nearby. One has a younger brother who snowboarded off a cliff as seen on TV. The young brother had no advance staff to map hazards, so he free-fell sixty feet and hit a rock with his head. That was earlier today. Surgery is now. I wait with these boys and share my anxiety over heroic measures and a system based on exclusion and obfuscation. The boys are more agreeable to the place, however, agreeing that surgery in two hours flat is a miracle, and anyone who sues this place or these doctors ought to be shot. They don't know who will pay for the younger brother's surgery, but by God he's in there having the top quarter of his brain removed, and the doctors are doing their level best. "Removed?"

"Yeah. It's the part you don't hardly use anyway."

"Ah." I think this system is designed for these boys and their brother, who live by faith and acceptance of what they're told. The mother arrives and embraces both boys. They grieve.

A family group on the far side enlarges on arrival of five more and two toddlers. The toddlers are released to wander the waiting room. Both drool garden slugs from their noses. One is taking a shit. The place reeks and wails. I wish everyone well and move out to the corridor with two chairs.

Hospital air feels stale, but the air in the corridor is at least breathable. I sit by the door leading to the patio reserved for smokers. It's seven o'clock, after hours, so the reception desk is unattended. I pick up the phone and press the second button down on the right, as instructed. I ask for Anne. I remind her who I am and ask for status. She says she'll find out. Call back in five minutes. I wait five minutes and call back. "They're just now inside," she says. "It's going well, on schedule. She's doing fine. They haven't yet exposed the clot or the aneurysm."

"On schedule? It's been three hours."

"They're very deliberate in there. That's what you want. Pre-op is at least an hour. I can tell you this, though: They say she was very peaceful going under the anesthesia."

"You mean more peaceful than most, or more peaceful than they expected?"

"They don't expect anything. They try to be ready. They see many reactions. Hers was very good."

"Well, thanks. I'll check back in a while."

"All right. Give them an hour or two."

"I'll try."

I ring off and sit. I wait and stare. I watch people come and go; they embrace with a shudder against fear and loss. The lament rises and falls. A very old woman counsels her family that someone must be here at all times now. I can't tell if she shares my apprehension on heroic measures, but I think not; I think she wants her husband to have company in his passing. Others simply meet outside to embrace and cry.

And here comes Stuey with a brown paper bag. I don't depend on a personal God for personal needs, yet I thank the spirits for their emissary. In the bag is a six-pack. I stand and lead the way to the smokers' exile. Outside I am humbled in realizing the value of company and cold beer. Stuey is full of life; this will take a few more hours, so why don't we go somewhere decent, like a bar.

I tell him I need to be here, and I pop another beer.

He shrugs and lights a joint.

I take it deep as a drowning man grabbing for any rope in reach, but you don't get "high" when you're pressed this low. Stuey rambles over a phase of his life he never mentioned but that I should know about, which was his brief career in anesthesiology. He took part in dozens of procedures like this one. Dozens. "It's a cakewalk, man. In and out. No sweat."

"You were an anesthesiologist?"

"Yeah, man. Well, I was going to be one. I scrubbed up with those guys."

"Why didn't you become one?"

He raises both palms like the Pope. "I was in it two years. The money's good, plenty nurses, but Christ, how can you adjust to this, day in and day out?" I nod. "Besides, I got an offer at Vamac. It worked out." Vamac is his current employer, where sales are good, but trends can be problematic. At least the current cycle is good, with positive indices and growth likely. His gab is tireless.

We go back inside. I'm freezing. He reassures me that a standard craniotomy is a simple tune-up, especially on a straight shot to the temporal lobe. "They just shave the head, cut the scalp, peel it back..."

"Please." We take our seats.

"No, really, cut the skull with this incredible little buzz saw. It only turns a sixteenth each way, like the saw they use to cut casts off, so they won't tear the soft tissue. Lift the brain flap, sponge the clot and it's done."

"They have to clip the aneurysm."

"Is that what they said? That's easy. Clip it off, set the skull piece back, sew her up and we have a few drinks."

"When were you exposed to this sort of thing?"

"Oh, hell, man, it's been twenty, twenty-three years."

"They clamp the skull piece back with titanium plates now."

"You're kidding."

I shake my head. "I don't know why they would use an unnatural material, except that maybe the anti-spasm drug they're giving her is a calcium-channel blocker, so the bone can't heal on its own."

"That's it! I remember; they used to have big problems with the skull piece mending into place."

I wonder what else he remembers. "They screw the plates into place."

"Much better. I'll tell you it's a weird trip down there. I hit the wall. I got used to carting the stiffs out. But after surgery was the worst, you know with the gore and shit."

"Do you mind?"

"No. But I gotta tell you what really did it for me. They had this guy in there, old guy, eighty-five or so. He's on the table and they got him splayed open like a road kill, and he dies. You know how the beep, beep, beep just goes beeeeeeeeep? I was moving some things around by the operating table, and this guy, I don't know if he was an orderly or a nurse or a doctor or what, but he figures out that the plasma bag is empty. That's why the old guy died. They always keep the next one hanging right there so they can make the change, you know, but they didn't make it and the old guy died, and this guy lunges for the plasma to make the change and maybe bring this old guy back. Who the hell knows? But he misses and just barely hits the new bag with a scalpel or something, and it breaks and sprays all over the damn place, and I'm right under it . . .

"Those guys . . . They just quit and walked out, and I have to sponge the old guy down and get rid of the scrubs and sheets and mop the floor and wheel the dead guy to the morgue. It was horrible."

"What were you, a cub anesthesiologist?"

"Yeah, kind of. It was completely different then. They played music in the OR and, you know, drugs were cool then. They can't pull that shit anymore."

"Mm. Another reason for getting out."

"I don't know. I'm telling you though; they do standard craniotomies three, four times a day. She'll be fine in no time."

"What about the mortality/morbidity disclosures they keep hosing me down with?"

"Fuck those guys. They're so scared of lawsuits they got the whole system turned around. They don't give a shit who they scare. They just want to cover their asses."

"Tell me this, Doctor, since you're the only medical staff here who might understand my particular situation."

"Yes?"

"Rachel and I enjoy recreational stimulants. Do we face compromise?"

"Nah! She'll get drunk easier is all. Probably enjoy sex more. They do after that view. That's why nurses are hot."

"Maybe the nurses are different now too."

"Yeah. I suppose. What a shame."

I check my watch. "It's eight-thirty. I'm going to check."

"They won't know anything."

"But they do." I call Anne. She asks me to call back in five minutes, which I do.

But she only says, "They're all the way in. It's going well. Give me an hour."

"Was I right?" Stuey asks.

I don't respond. So he insists we have all the time in the world for a bar and a few martinis. I insist that I can't. So we go outside for two more beers. He won't shut up, reviewing prospects for the unbelievable business that's coming his way. He says huge volume isn't even a variable anymore, because the economy is so hot these guys want it right now and don't even peep when he jacks the price twelve points, as long as he can deliver now.

Maybe he sees my inattention. He shifts gears to our upcoming scooter rides over the mountains, just around the corner in April and May and then, look out, summertime. I smile, wishing it were summer now. We remember the glory times, but they too go to murmurs and then silence and the shivers set in.

A few minutes before ten I call Anne again and call her back in five minutes. "They're closing her up," she says. "It went very well. She's not even intubated. She was, but she did so well, they removed it." Intubation delivers forced air for those who can't continue breathing, and it prevents constriction, likely from reverse peristalsis. I feel like I'm on the mend, thinking of reverse peristalsis instead of puking. Who knows? If the throat constricts anyway they go quickly to tracheotomy and an air hose through the neck. Oh, it's not a pretty place. At least Rachel was spared that part of it.

"Can they tell yet about the . . . morbidity?"

"We think there wasn't any. You won't know for sure until she's out of recovery. You'll want to be there. We want her to recognize you and speak coherently."

"You mean in a sentence?"

"A sentence would be ideal. Let's see. She should be up there by eleven-thirty or midnight, right on schedule. The surgeon is looking for you in the OR waiting room."

"He's done?"

"Yes. Closing is rudimentary."

"I thought I was in the OR waiting room. They told me to wait in Two West."

"No. Go downstairs. I'll call him and tell him you'll meet him there."

"Thank you, Anne." I set the phone down and feel my face respond to the lateral gravities of joy and non-restraint. Stuey hovers near and now sees the news on me. "They're done," I say. "They're closing her up.

She didn't die. And no apparent morbidity." He shakes his head with a smile of his own and begins another silly rant on I-told-you-so. But he stops because I am breaking down, heaving from inside out as the dark spirit rails in disappointment. I am gently pressed and then heavily moved as great chunks of glacier overhanging the sea for way too long fall away in thundering release. I join the lament.

My friend hugs and rocks me. I cannot speak but rather spew the grief of days and nights and in equal measure the fear of years. "It's okay," he says.

But it's not.

"It's okay. It's okay," he insists, but I've had it up to here and way beyond. "It's okay. She's okay. Hey. Hey. Hey."

I don't know that the dam ever burst on such a reservoir. It gushes forth and gushes again. It flows in torrents until the flood-gates can gain a purchase and slowly close, until nothing remains but puddles. "Okay, I'm done. I'm okay," I say, wiping my face, breathing deep, gathering my manly self and standing straight. He nods, not as spent as I am but significantly removed from a minute ago, and we're off to meet the wizard.

Lawrence of Neurology is just a guy like us, of course, but it helps to see him loose, removed from his suit and tie and formal demeanor. He wears sleeveless scrubs and a skullcap. He shakes my hand like a good sport after a match, as if now we can let our friendship show. He says it went very well, according to plan with no surprises, and she should recover to a hundred percent in a short time.

"No debilitation?" I ask.

He delivers the tight-lipped smile, as if legal defense is understood between us. I think he means to convey that Rachel is past the risk of morbidity, maybe, but who can say? Certainly not him.

Stuey asks how big was the clot. Lawrence is relieved with a question of fact, free of conjecture; he brightens, turning to Stuey, and says, "Golf ball—well, actually closer to a lemon."

"Big lemon?"

Lawrence smiles again; how big is a lemon? Then he nods. "It was very big."

"Any trouble sponging it out?"

Lawrence has no time for shop talk with a fiberboard salesman. So he walks away, telling us over his shoulder, "No. Most of it comes out in a clump anyway."

We go up to the ninth floor and back to the ICU corridor to wait for another hour or two. The two guys with the younger brother are there as well, waiting. We review snowboarding, medivac helicopters, surgery, litigation and the system, but we keep it simple, avoiding morbidity. They want only the safe return of the younger brother to the construction crew. I think theirs is a world without end.

We sit. We wait.

We wait more.

A few minutes before midnight the elevator opens. We sit up as we have done every time it opens, but this is it, two nurses in front, two in back, easy, easy, gently over the bumps and out. I fear the view of my woman drenched in carnage, but I step quickly up.

Stuey stands beside me. The attendants pause briefly, and we are struck with a sight I will never forget. Rachel is still wired to many leads. She is wrapped in blankets with her head swathed in gauze over the top and around the sides so that only her face is showing. She radiates as if lit from inside, more alive than I've ever seen a person, effusing color and energy, brightness and warmth—and strength and movement even though she lies serenely still. Her lips are moist, her cheeks glowing. Angels hover overhead in a swirl and a song.

Yes—this one is as tough to explain as anything I've ever known. You can't talk about angels without inviting the easy discount, without sounding like a hopeless romantic who hopes against hope against what has come to pass. But this too is as real as the fear and darkness; here is a vision. Here the ether palpitates in rare articulation. I see spirits engaged in movement, raising their voice in a harmony more deafening than the silence of the canyons. They have no lyric, no arms or legs or harps or long white beards. They have fish tails and they swirl in gaudy colors. They have cat whiskers, briefly, and hooked beaks and wing feathers. They loll their tongues and wag their tails. They're watchful, busy and alert, ready to rise against intruders.

They're only smoke or fog. Or maybe something in my eye is refracting the light just so, breaking it down to what my heart wants most to see. These spirit visions are likely nothing but a distraction reflecting the personal order of an original animal nut.

Yet Stuey sees something too.

"Holy shit," he whispers.

"Oh, yes," I agree.

9

---◆◆---

Time for Service!

We are quickly waved off and waved back. We must sit and wait till she comes to the surface. She should regain consciousness soon, or she could drift indefinitely deeper and farther away. If she fails to blink or mutter she'll be dragged to the surface by injection. I cringe at every flex of the heavy hand, but the system is built on data, and the numbers are deemed the ultimate truth. Into the last phase of this gauntlet, our self-evaluation as healthful people living significantly above the lowest common denominator is incidental. Human response to radical drugs is the object of absolute belief, of faith that we will live and/or die within a 4% margin of error. We can only sit and wait. And shut up.

In a few minutes I'm called back. She's in a private room with walls and a door. What a relief. But this place and the system have made me tentative at every turn. Are they treating us better because our odds are now longer? That's cynical, possibly paranoid, what a walk down the street might feel like after a mugging. Never mind. I want her to open her eyes and see me, optimistic as a Rotarian. I plant a smile on my face to better solicit a sentence with a subject and verb, period.

She barely breaks the surface and can't stay afloat. She squirms slightly like a worm on concrete near the end of the struggle. The radiance is still on her, but it also twists with overlapping layers of pain, with fear of death and worse, of mutilation or debilitation. I sense the struggle is above her and in her, between the dark other and the others I witnessed a few minutes ago. She opens her eyes. She stares at me, not with recognition but in disbelief, as if to ask, *How could you?* She seems heartbroken, grieved at a loss of trust, at what I caused to happen. I stretch my smile and tell her how proud I am. I tell her how strong she is, how well it went, how well she's doing, how soon we'll be home.

She reaches to touch my face or maybe she sees something else, so I lean close. She feels my cheek, but this is not for love. She can't see right, can't find my depth, can't be certain who I am. She lets her hand fall and rolls to one side as the hope and desire in me ebbs to zero. She moans, "I'm so unhappy."

Oh, God. I am happy now, though my smile twists in the grasp of sadness—sadness reverberates from my usually happy mate. Tension melts when she speaks, subject and verb and all the rest. I tell her to rest easy; I'll be back in the morning first thing. She says, "Take your time. Go have some fun." That's three sentences, and she knows it's me, though we hang in space and time like rags on a bucket.

Soon she slips under, giving in to the stone tied to her ankles, sinking again to morphine dreams. This will piss her off; she doesn't like pharmaceuticals. But I let it pass and let the drug flow, because I frankly think she's still in denial. Maybe I am too. Things seem different now, as if we're coming out.

The hospital provides pamphlets on what ails you or a loved one. Statistics for morbidity and mortality remain consistent, and each is written to the lowest denominator of comprehension skills. Each pamphlet focuses on specific needs of the most debilitating potentials. Between these lines is the ghost of mortality. Short of that is severe handicap and redundancy, so you can't say we didn't warn you.

I read of the devastation that will change my daily life and that of everyone around me. But I don't read too far, for I'm sensitive to toxins and can fortunately smell them before swallowing. One noted physician feels that in the entire subarachnoid outing, surgery is the easiest part of all. Challenges of extreme potential come next. I think he presumes the ease of surgery to be a function of coma and/or anesthesia; the system can more easily process an unconscious patient—damn. I check myself against negativity once more, imagining Bre'r Bear strolling down a country road whistling Zippety Do Da.

I repress the negative potential. We survive and soon we'll thrive. The physician in the pamphlet is meant to ease the family into post-op, his message apparently distilled by legal counsel to careful wording. I don't want to be knee-jerk to every helpful effort coming our way, but I've been conditioned to be on guard.

"What are you reading? Let's go."

I agree. Stuey wants a bar, a wild one where we can really celebrate. I also appreciate his challenge, more than that of the brochures, but he is also dismissed. "I've had very little sleep and not much to eat the last few days. I can't."

"Well. Okay. Let's go back to the office then. We can stop at Larry's for a barbecued chicken. That'll be better. Have a few beers. Get high. You still got some of that apple brandy?" I nod. Larry's is closed, so we stop at Quality Foods, open 24 hours.

In no time we're swilling beer and brandy, firing joints, eating greasy chicken with two hands and reviewing the bogus taste and engineering of the Harley Davidson designers. We both anticipate trading up in another season. I may ponder BMW or Victory or anything less wasteful and with better handling. Stuey agrees—but forlornly, because he's stuck in an image. In that small world he thinks he'll go ahead with chrome wheels. Because, frankly, he's tired of running spokes and tube tires on the open road, where a flat could shut him down and leave him stranded. "Who needs that?" He shifts quickly and jumps to my desk, grabbing my binoculars with his greasy hands and scanning the building a block over. "There! Look!" He's found a female and is certain she's in a bedroom, where she will undoubtedly take her clothes off. I pour us another short round of apple brandy. "Look at this," he implores.

I drink and tell him, "I think Madonna could walk in here with her thumb up her pussy, and I couldn't care less."

He laughs. He can't share my indifference but appreciates the imagery. "Her thumb?" he asks, moving his fingers in a test pattern near his pussy. "I *guess* her thumb would work."

I laugh too. "It's a figure of speech." I need peace and rest. I'm amazed again at how quickly life restores itself; with basic needs fulfilled. I have fed. I need sleep. But I take the binocs he hands me and I watch the woman across the way. She's not in a bedroom. She's having a drink with a man. I tell him it's unbelievable what she's doing now, dropping to her knees and, no, it can't be . . . Stuey laughs, rolling another joint. Finally, I'm catching on to why he's here, to engage in foolish behavior and facilitate my high. I've suffered overexposure to mortality/morbidity, so I accept his guidance now in cold, clinical light, as if his silly antics are integral to rehab. Besides, his challenge seems only moderate with no potential. I try my best to go along with his system.

Soon we both tire and turn in to keep from passing out. Stuey will sleep on a futon he happened to bring along. It's down in his car. He has only to shag it, unless of course I want him to put his underpants on backwards and lay down with me. I laugh, but I'm already on the sofa, wondering why he planned to stay over all along, as if he knows something else about the cakewalk we've just been through.

But I only care for the very few minutes it takes to fall asleep. I'm out by the time he's back up. I sleep a solid six hours, my longest nap in days, and awake marginally rested if not refreshed. Stuey rises slowly, insisting on a good breakfast, because a man has to eat. He knows a place, and we soon face ungodly mounds of eggs over hash browns alongside ham and toast. I eat slowly. He engorges till he puts his napkin on the counter and says it's time to go drop the kids off at the pool.

"What kids? What pool?" But he's off. Watching the grease congeal, I wonder what the day and night just past would have been like in solitude. I don't doubt my survival, but I would have drunk and smoked less, slept more fitfully and eaten nothing. Doctor Stuey is back in two minutes. "Just that quick?"

"Yeah. It's a miracle. This place is great."

I excuse myself to make my bid for greatness. I realize that Stuey is an original pain in the ass and a friend in need. I dispense with fear and morbidity and ease on back to the counter, where Stuey is having more coffee and a smoke. "Yeah, you're right. This place is great. I have to go now."

"I'm coming with you. Okay? I want to see her."

We go in two cars, because I'm staying for the shift. My car bongs for ten seconds and shuts up. I haven't listened to the radio in three days, or four. I turn it on to the Byrds singing *Don't Fear the Reaper*. It assures me that forty thousand men and women every day . . . That was thirty years ago, when it was only forty thousand people dying daily. I flip to jazz, not smooth jazz, but the straight-ahead stuff that helps some people reconcile the contradictions all around us. I'm one of those jazz fans. A tenor sax won't explain the complexities of life, but it speaks to the beautiful effort we must make in resolving things, in syncopating the challenges with a few swinging eighth notes on the way.

Up again in the ICU, Stuey says he'll wait. She'll want to see me first.

I enter slowly. Her eyes are closed. I ascertain her breathing then pick up the new chart near the computer. On top is a printed form issued post-op, a multiple-choice series of questions with a few fill-in-the blanks. The new profile is:

47 yo ♀ L temporal 3 cm

INTRAPERENCLLYMAL HSURATEMA

L MCA Bifurcation Aneurysm

- ALERT *Anxious Uncooperative*
- Responds to voice
- Responds to pain
- Unresponsive

She opens her eyes but doesn't smile as I finish reading. I sense further symptoms of displeasure with lingering distrust. She displays what is profiled in longhand as *anxious* and *uncooperative*. I'm present with moral support, beginning with my opinion that anyone free of anxiety and willing to cooperate in this house of shrinks and disclaimers would require another box to check:

◆ Bona fide android.

But she underscores my own culpability with a headshake and another complete sentence, "I wish I hadn't done that."

"We had no choice," I remind her. "It's over now. You're doing great."

"It's not over. Look at me." I look. She is wired like a control center, pierced with needles leading to narrow diameter plastic tubing festooned and tangled. She complains of a searing pain in her back and a splitting headache. I don't laugh as I assure her that discomfort at this point is a no-brainer, that pain and a headache are to be expected after cerebral surgery. She doesn't laugh either, so I don't press.

From the top of her head, out of the gauze rises a six-inch steel spike connected to a bundle of leads and plastic tubing twisted in a bunch and running to her monitor. These are to measure brain pressure for the critical period of seventy-two hours after surgery. I will ask many people many times what will happen in the event of cranial swelling. I am given mutters and mumbles but no answer, maybe because the team is tired of my need to know, or maybe because the answer could be construed as libelous. I let it slide, and I repress further assessment of extreme potential. I will work with the team, as I'm able to do so, defending my mate's right to autonomy if not peace. I pause here, as I would come to do many times in the months ahead, to consider the overwhelming need upon us to get along, even as society rears its ugly face. I squelch my natural resistance to being treated this way, and I succeed. Chronic repression can lead to psychosis in the long term, but for the moment it helps prioritize the issues at hand.

Her forearms are pierced with many needles. They dangle from veins near arteries in both wrists. She is bruised with more yellow and purple than a hurricane sky—both wrists to both elbows. The right side of her neck is swollen like a bladder and seeps viscous ooze. The skin on that side of her neck looks like a goiter, dead and yellow, slumped like melted wax. From this misshapen, syrupy mess comes the gang valve with its many leads and a few more leads from valve splitters alongside. This neck apparatus has been re-sutured into place, but its sheer weight tugs at the flesh. It's difficult to look at. She sees the difficulty in me, and her facial expression sinks further. Then I see that the horribly dead, sloughed skin is not really skin but the packing tape holding the hardware and veins into her neck, to keep all the stuff from plopping out. "Oh, hell," I say. "It's tape—not skin but tape."

She feels it with her hand, pressing and crying out in pain, "God."

"What?"

"Feel this." She tugs at her gown. I assist. Between her crotch and thigh is a hacked, purple lump as big as an egg—the femoral artery. I touch it, rock solid. She cries again.

"Sorry."

"No. My back."

"Can you roll over? I can help your back."

She whines and whimpers as she struggles through the tangle of tubing and leads, pushing through the pain, because she knows of the magic in my hands. I pull her gown up and see the punctures left by the spinal taps. They're a quarter inch across and thick, like rocks are bulging from under the skin. I won't touch these but put my palms on her back, higher up. She's burning up. I move carefully, leading the heat and pain out where I can. She mutters regret once more, wishing she'd never come here, wishing her life had ended, if that was meant to be, without this nightmare finale.

In a few minutes I pull her gown back down and cover her. She's sleeping. The radiance is gone. Now she looks beat and broken, body and soul. She looks beyond the pale of mortal concern, quite willing to stop this process, if not by going home then by going beyond.

I walk into the hall and ask the charge nurse for our nurse. Our nurse is Leah again, and I ask what's on the agenda for today. I fear a downturn in vital function that may warrant medical urgency, what the system will not call heroic, but I anticipate the heroic motivation. I fear it, with its TV reality, its voltage and drama. Of course that's just me being cynical and difficult once again, as necessary.

Yet I must consider prospects for more critical needs, for re-entry, with Rachel's scalp peeled back again, the skull unscrewed, another spinal tap or two and some fiddling around because the repairman couldn't get it right the first time. I don't want to suspect that a few adjustments will be warranted to enhance the database but can't help it. A few more tests could be covered by the insurance and justified in the pursuit of data critical to the great experiment, in which the system will be further proven. She's so healthy, and a case could be made for shoring up the mean. This sounds irrational, but I am accountable to my mate and determined to defend her, even before the trouble has a chance to begin.

Though I felt relief only a few hours ago, I sense a new arrival, or perhaps a regression. I teeter on a brink between will and default. Sleep can alleviate physical fatigue but not spiritual fatigue. Years ago we agreed, Rachel and I, what we would do when the ball came to us rather than waiting to think it over and losing the play. We would know what to do for each other because we shared an outlook on life and death, because death is unavoidable and in some circumstances should not be prolonged or unduly agonized.

This may not be one of those circumstances, but the unavoidable feeling is that it may. We agreed in a brief but sobering session to do the same for each other in regard to plugging and unplugging. We went for drinks and danced up a sweat after that strategy session, to forget what would come to pass, to drench the inevitable in oblivion.

We agreed to facilitate passage with peace. We will impart dignity to the space around us, surrounding ourselves with what we love rather than beeping machinery working off a heavy debt service and in fact losing money unless plugged in. Nurse Leah assures me that the surgery will not be repeated in any event. The brain will not be exposed again, nor will the screws be re-torqued or the incision tampered with in any way. This assurance is a relief and is key to our needs, so fragile seems Rachel's connection to life.

No, the rough part is over, I am told, even if she suffers spasm (stroke) or seizure—over, that is, unless her brain swells. After one last angiogram, Nurse Leah says, we will face no more invasiveness, except of course on our privacy and rationale. She adds this as support and understanding.

"When are we scheduled for the angiogram?"

Leah checks her watch. "About twenty minutes. But first, we have to—"

"No. That can't happen."

"It has to happen. We need a baseline for her pressure and flow so we can measure her progress over the next few days."

"No."

"We can't know if she's failing without it."

"No. You'll kill her."

"I'll call the neurosurgeon on duty. It's his decision."

"You're a great nurse, Leah," I tell her. She pauses for rote patronization—she's heard it before. "But don't ever forget whose decision it is. It's not his decision."

She puts a hand on my arm. "I'm sorry. I'll get him."

The surgeon on duty is young but also tired, at the end of a long and difficult shift. He doesn't stop nodding when Nurse Leah tells him of my concern. He stops nodding only when I correct her by saying that I'm not merely concerned; there will be no angiogram. He breaks into the neurological, clinical and critical needs for another angiogram, without which all the effort so far may be for naught. I reach deep for patience, and I tell him, "You have her wired to ninety-seven vital functions. You can tell her pressure and flow and rate and tempo and altitude and specific gravity at a glance. I'm telling you, and you need to hear me, that Rachel is a tediously happy person, who now verges on emotional and spiritual failure, and that's why people die in hospitals."

To my amazement, Leah is nodding now.

"Not one of those machines in there can give you a level of depression. I'm telling you it's deep, and it's the emotion most often preceding death. We're in dangerous territory. You will leave her alone. I have spoken before witnesses. There will be no angiogram."

He shakes his head in a uniquely forlorn way, different than that of a wise man facing resistance but more of a young doctor denied standard protocol. He's worked very hard for years and all night long to learn and to serve. We know this. We feel this. We recognize his stature.

I saw the same look back in Bremerton, presented with a consent form that allowed us to decline the medivac helicopter.

"Listen," he says. "We do this—"

"You're not doing it this time."

"I have an idea," Leah says. "I think she's upset because of, you know, all the IV leads and bruises and the antenna, and they left the dressing on her head, and the tape. I think I can eliminate some of the twelve leads. Some are redundant, and I can use some of the others for multiple functions. We might get her down to six leads."

The young doctor looks professionally skeptical, but he is pre-empted by the old fool, as I chime in, "Yes. Less is more. Let's proceed."

Leah cannot take initiative without approval from a "superior," who gives me the look and follows up with conviction that I am now putting my wife's life in jeopardy. I've heard it before in many forms. He is trying to close the deal on guilt, so that we may move beyond our intuition and instinct to data-based protocol proven effective to within four percent margin of error.

"You can have your angiogram," I tell him, "But later, after she has a few hours or maybe a day to regain her composure." I will not tell him that the numbers are compelling or that I am driven solely by instinct. You give these guys an inch, next thing you know it's the miracle mile, bring on the defibrillators.

In minutes Rachel is relieved of six of her twelve leads. Leah strips her down and removes big patches of postal tape smothering her pores, along with patches of congealed wound dressing that look like dirty glue, maybe two square feet from Rachel's chest, back and arms. To my amazement, Rachel sits up with a smile. "I want this stuff off my head. It's really closing in on me."

"Okay. We can do that," Leah chirps, which brings further relief to Rachel but chills me with anticipation.

"You're going to take the bandage off?" I ask.

"Yeah. We don't need it. It's only on there so you won't get scared."

"Yeah, well . . ."

Leah deftly unwraps the battered head. I reach again for an immovable smile and hold it there, because I am scrutinized like a mirror. "Tell me," she says. "What do I look like?"

Her head is shaved on the left side. A horseshoe-shaped scar runs from the top, center of her forehead, back and around and down to just beside the left ear. The scar is about ten inches long, just as the doctor had advised. Zigzagging a tight pattern around the bend are fifty-six stitches. I shrug. "You look like you. What are you supposed to look like?"

She frowns and demands, "Tell me what I look like!" I see the monitor as her pressure and pulse climb ten points in the next two seconds.

"You look like Queen Elizabeth with a face lift by Dr. Frankenstein. What difference does it make?"

"Give me my mirror. I want to see." She is quickly weak and fragile, her voice quivering.

"No, no. Why bother yourself? You had surgery a few hours ago. Let it rest."

"Give. Me. My. Mirror."

Fortunately she has only a two-inch compact, so she can't take in the full gore. The wound has oozed what appear to be four or five egg yolks. Leah assures me this is only more suture dressing. She removes most of it, peeling it off. Worse yet is the steel spike with more plastic tubing coming out the top of her head. Nurse Leah explains, "This measures brain pressure. We call it your antenna."

"It looks more like a dipstick than an antenna," I say, hardly intending to compound the difficulty, but I feel difficult, more so than usual.

"Yes, well, antenna sounds nicer. We can get rid of it in seventy-two hours. You're doing unbelievably well."

Rachel looks pained and incredulous. "I am?"

"Are you kidding? You're awake, talking, moving around."

"I feel better with that stuff off. But I don't feel good. Look at me. I want the rest of this stuff off me."

"You will have it off. Every last bit and soon. I can take this one off, too. You're not even draining." Leah fiddles with another lead, as if knowing precisely which strand of spaghetti wants attention. This one runs to the left temporal lobe or the back end or somewhere in the tangle. I don't ask what could be draining, nor can I watch too closely as another plastic check valve on the end of a turkey baster is pulled from a soft area of the skull.

"*Yellow matter custard*," I murmur. "*Bleeding from a dead dog's eye.*"

"What are you saying?" Rachel gasps.

"It's just glue," I say. "And a distraction. You remember the Beatles' song, *I Am the Walrus*. *Coo coo catchou. Everybody smoke pot. Everybody smoke pot.*"

"You need a CAT scan," she says.

Nurse Leah leaves with the mess. Rachel preens hopelessly like a cat after a losing fight, smoothing here, straightening there, but failing to hide the terrific beating she has taken. I take the opportunity to explain the need for an additional . . . well, er, uh . . . procedure. What we need is not a CAT scan for me but one more angiogram for her, but not today, or at least not this morning, so she can have time to rest. And after that, we are honestly and truly on the mend, no more procedures no matter what. And that's no shit.

"Let's get it over with," she says.

I turn to tell the head neuro to hurry up or I'll sue, but I check myself, my humor is so often ill-advised and in this case it feels wrong to me too, which may be grounds for optimism on seeing the light at last. But what light can possibly deny a sense of humor?

This question must wait as I remember our old friend Stuey outside. I re-enter Rachel's room to say that Stuey is here to visit her.

"He's here?"

I nod.

"I can't see anyone like this."

I feel foolish, bringing guests to see the gore and prolonging the inevitable angiogram. I think I should have slept late.

"He just wants to say hello."

"No. I'm not ready."

I walk out and tell Stuey she's not feeling well and doesn't want company. He understands, asking gently if she's doing well. "I think so. It's hard to say. She's depressed. And pissed at me."

He laughs. "You just have to splain it to her." He wants to know if I want to join him for a cruise around town, to check a few things out. I tell him no, I need some rest. I'll hang out here for a while. He assures me that hanging out here is cool. He'll call later. Maybe we'll do something.

I find Leah and tell her we can proceed anytime with the angiogram. She says we now must wait until this afternoon; the morning schedule filled up. I don't care, but I wonder what other industry enjoys such a market response. Why do they press so urgently, when another customer is ready? Well, I never doubted the sincerity of the place, I just don't take to a process so critical to my future but that has no place for my thoughts.

Back in the curtained space Rachel is again napping. I sit and stare. The curtain soon opens on a food server. In the chafing dish is stuffed ravioli in smegma sauce with fat globules drifting in the littorals. I only think this. I don't speak. I don't have to: Rachel opens her eyes and nearly swoons. I cover the dish and set it out in the hall. She says she couldn't eat if she had to. She encourages me to eat it, so it won't be wasted. I mumble that we must waste it to keep it from wasting me. Her eyes close on my clever retort, and in moments she's sound asleep. I ponder the relative character of waste. She'll have to eat soon.

In a while she wakens feebly and asks what kind of drug is going into her vein. She feels lightheaded. I get Nurse Leah, who smiles and says, "That's morphine, honey."

Rachel struggles up. "Morphine? I don't want morphine. Which one is it?" Her fingers feel the many lines plumbed into her veins. She is poised, ready to pluck the morphine lead from either arm. Or is it one of those in her calves? Or her neck?

"Wait! I'll turn it off. No more morphine."

"Yuck. No wonder I feel bad."

I tell her I'm going to the grocery for a chicken and some vegetables. I'll make her a hearty broth. How does that sound?

"Yuck. I can't eat."

"It won't be ready for a few hours."

"Fine. Go. And take your time. Have some fun. You don't need to be here."

You don't need to be here. I wonder where I need to be besides there or running all over hell for some goddamn chicken soup. The car won't stop bonging. It seems louder now, or maybe it's wearing me down. The lights have spread from the console data panel to the dash to the emergency message center. *Time for Service! Service Now!* I press the buttons in variable sequence. I would punch the buttons, but that would be foolish. Shooting the buttons would be more foolish and expensive but it has a definite appeal, but I have no gun. I stew, until realizing that this could be the perfect time to get the car serviced. Once we're out of the hospital, it could be weeks before I get back over. These bells and lights are telling me where I need to be, if only I can listen. I make an appointment for the afternoon. The woman in service says, "You know we'll have to keep it overnight."

I tell her they can bury it for all I care.

Oh my, she says.

I apologize, restating my position. "I don't mind if you keep it overnight is what I meant to say."

"Do you need a rental?"

"No. I can cab it."

"If you don't mind my saying, you sound very stressed."

"I'm a bit stressed, yes. We've had a . . . medical emergency."

"You have a coupon in your glove box good for a free day's rental. I'll set it up. I don't want you to be without a car. Can you be here by three?"

"Yes, I can." I speak conspicuously nicely now, wondering how she moved me so easily from angst to gratitude. "Yes. I . . . appreciate your . . ."

"Don't you worry. We'll take care of you."

Who'd a thunk it; car people? I proceed to the grocery, because industry is good. I'm relieved but not pleased. We're on our way out of the Valley of the Shadow of Death, but it still feels like a slog through a very long dream. We're past the worst of it but not yet in the clear. My mate is on the mend, but tension lingers. I think the tension is mostly mine, and I wonder why it's become unmanageable.

Well, the car won't shut up or leave me be. The little bell rings and lights flash on each start. Wail while you can, you little . . . car, because it won't be long now—I laugh, perhaps getting at the root of what ails me. It's self-induced, kind of, a minor crazing brought on by stress. But I think I have everything to pursue a simple, productive task, and making chicken soup should be a positive process. But I have no Thermos, and coming out again for a Thermos for the soup, after returning to the office to prepare the soup, could be negative. As it is I must chase a tune-up and then hurry back to the front, where I may be chided again for my concern or told that the idea of soup makes her want to puke. At least I'm sorting and planning ahead. I'll stop at U-Sav-Mor for a Thermos. On the way I call Nurse Leah. "How is Rachel doing?"

"I know it's hard for you to accept, but she really is doing terrific. You wouldn't believe how well she's doing. You would if you could see some of the others coming through that procedure."

"Good. I wish she wasn't so depressed."

"That's normal."

"Leah. Depression isn't normal."

"Oh yes it is, if you've been through what she's been through. She's on her way to angio. She'll be there for a while. She's fine."

"When will we know about the angiogram?"

"This afternoon. But it's not a test. It's a baseline. They won't go in again."

"Yes. I heard that. Okay. I'll see you soon."

"I'm off at three. Chin up."

Yes. Chin up. Make the soup. But the U-Sav-Mor is under remodel. Thermos inventory is in back, packed and inaccessible. "We can't sell you one if we can't get to them."

"I feel confident that we can get to them. Let's go unpack one."

"Oh, no. We can't do that." Apparent here to the casual observer and the store clerk is my insistence. I could explain motivation shouldn't need to with inventory on hand and a sale waiting to be made. Should it?

I stew, and the clerk says, "You can try City Market. They have Thermoses." I look out the window. "It's easy," he says. "Straight down this street, three blocks."

I go three blocks down and cut over two blocks and come back one, because Bell is one-way from 4th Avenue eastward. I double park at City Market and go in but "No. We have no Thermos Bottles. We do. But we don't. Not now. Not right now. Later, maybe, but not right now. I mean ..."

"God damn it." I think the young female behind the counter is neither fluent nor lucid, and my expletive is another symptom, because this feels like a conspiracy—not an organized conspiracy but the random conspiracy of the world we live in, the world that doesn't work much of the time.

"Hey," a man says, stepping forward. "What's with you and a Thermos?"

"My wife hasn't eaten in five days. I mean she has, but only intravenously."

"She's in the hospital?"

"Yes, and she can't eat what they serve."

He stares, perhaps recalling hospital fare. He turns to a shelf and turns back with a Thermos, early 50's vintage in metallic green with chrome trim. "Here. Take mine. Wait a minute. I'll rinse it for you."

"I can't take your Thermos."

"Why not? She's hungry. She's got to eat. Besides, I want a new one. I been thinking about it. I'll rinse it."

"No. I'll rinse it." I accept the old Thermos. "Thank you."

"You're welcome."

"Yeah."

"Hey. Good luck."

"Thanks. I ..." I'm stuck.

"Go feed your wife."

I go. The old Thermos is worn like me, dented and dinged. It's been aground and sideswiped, but it doesn't rattle. The grocer used two big hose clamps to affix a drawer pull vertically for easy carrying, and my initials are scratched onto the side of this Thermos, as if sooner or later

I was meant to have it. I feel better with a task back on track and better yet, sensing the grocer as a guy throwing a lifeline. It feels odd to be elated over an old Thermos. But the times are raw and testy. My mate is still adrift in heavy seas, and the line I want to throw feels too short. Well, enough of tangling lines and stormy imagery. My inclement disposition should be temporary. I think Leah would agree.

So I wait under cloudy skies. The fog rolls in and makes no difference.

The broth simmers. A chicken, potatoes, celery, tomatoes, leeks, carrots, parsley, garlic, cilantro, lemon juice, olive oil and light soy. I eat. It's too pungent but so am I. I dilute with water, fill the cleaned Thermos and head out in the afternoon. She hasn't eaten. What if she's not hungry? What if she's famished? What else can I do but take the soup? Am I wrong to wonder what I'll do, where I'll live and what changes I'll make, if . . . But enough of that. Nurse Leah said we're on the mend.

The service woman at the dealership leans in and holds the set button on my dashboard for four seconds. The ringing stops. What a fool I've been. She wants to know what happened and how things are. I tell her, and she shares her own adventure in non-response. She says, "They took my mother last October." She said her mother got to the hospital with unusual but mild symptoms, so the medical staff put her mother under general anesthesia for "observation." The medical staff then proceeded to exploratory surgery in pursuit of something vague. Then they wagged their heads and said nothing more could be done, because the mother was dead. "They said they didn't know why." I hope there's more here than meets the ear, yet I feel relieved to hear that I'm not the only crazy person out there.

We commiserate briefly on the roughshod medical system, and I go. The car rental shuttle is waiting. She says the medical staff would not talk to her. They acknowledged her but said they didn't have the time before, during and after the death. She only wishes for five minutes more, so she could say goodbye to her mother, who would have loved a farewell. "I think they botched it," she says, tears flowing. "I think they botch it on a regular basis and act dumb to avoid, you know, the consequences. And they didn't even let me say goodbye."

I may be the first person she's told. I touch her and feel a pain greater than my own, unresolved since October. I take her in for a hug, perhaps the same hug given me only yesterday, and there we stand, two people sharing a lifeline—or maybe it's only enough flotsam to keep us afloat. It works.

I tell her they're a tough bunch; you can't hate them, but you can't relax either. I share my view of a Norman Rockwell tableau of them, standing around in surgical scrubs, blushing and shuffling their feet. One is kicking the dirt and another is punching the air. They're strewn with scalpels and needles, stethoscopes, surgical tubing and suture thread, little saws, forceps, gloves, masks and miles of plastic tubing. Splattered with blood and guts like ragamuffins after a good romp in the gore, they smile sheepishly; they're the best, but they can be naughty too. The title is *Win Some, Lose Some.*

I can't be certain she appreciates my humor or knows Norman Rockwell. I don't explain things, because she appreciates my position, which is her position. "I'll pray for you," she sputters.

The shuttle driver is young, early twenties. In the white shirt and narrow tie of a shuttle driver, he grins with official goodwill, helping this car-rental experience to be a good one. We wait on another passenger who says he'll be right there; he's almost finished. He pecks at the keyboard on his laptop computer. He holds his chin and thinks. He hits more keys, and so on.

"Are we supposed to wait for this?" I ask, as the last guy begins his deliberate exit, three minutes worth, because he still has e-mail in his outbox, and it must go out, because it's very important. I think it's okay, because after a few more minutes he and I will never need to meet again.

He sits up front and asks the driver how many seats this vehicle has, and if this is the biggest SUV out there. The driver says ten seats, but Ford has a model that is the largest sport utility vehicle ever made, unless someone came along with a bigger one. The laptop guy says he's familiar with the big Ford and how it got backlash from the environmentalists, because it gets only seven miles to the gallon. He thinks the jumbo unit is great, and if people buy it, that proves its greatness. "If the environmentalists had their way, there wouldn't be any cars."

I'm an environmentalist. Cars, power lines, franchise foods, the death of nature and overpopulation get my goat. So do people insensitive to these things or the urgency of others. He's blind to what I see, so I lean forward, avoiding my personal shortcoming to the extent that I'm able. I ask, "What would we have if you had your way?" He ignores me, so I ask again, "What?"

"Hey! If someone wants to buy it!"

"If someone wants to buy pictures of your parents having sexual intercourse, should you sell them?"

"That's different," he mutters, and we ease off, repressing personal demons and images of his parents fucking. He looks out the window; who needs a lecture from a maniac? At the rental car place I let him go first.

Then it's my turn. "Hi! I'm Lisa, your service representative! Let's walk around your car to be sure!"

The car is a del Fuego, and looks like a go-kart with a sheet metal wrapping. It sounds like an eggbeater, and it rattles.

"A del Fuego. It sounds like something Elmer Fudd would dwive. I mean drive. We don't need to walk awound it."

"Please." She insists, so I walk around the little car behind her. She wears high heels and a tight skirt and lipstick. She carries a clipboard and keeps smiling, glancing back at me.

"It looks like a nice car. I think I'm going to love it."

She hands me the keys and says, "Have a nice day."

It feels like what we've come to, and soon I'm on my way in a two-by-two that can go fifty downhill. But it's a bumpy road on a bumpy day, and I anticipate further challenge up the road at the ICU, both personal and culinary. This is love and what love comes to. With luck, this time will soon be a memory, what we came to and passed through.

The little car's radio is preset to Christian stations and one station with elevator music. *A Man and A Woman* comes on—*baaaa daaa daaa*

da-da-da-da-da, baa daa daa da-da-da-da-da. The movie came out in
'66 when I was still a kid but felt much older, and anything French or
Italian seemed sophisticated. So were skinny ties and swingers.

I ponder a new movie for modern times, *A Man and A Woman Part
II* about this hyperkinetic health-nut woman who has an aneurysm and
her husband with floating hostility who wanders the earth while his wife
is in the ICU.

The idea makes me smile. I'd go see that movie. I'd have popcorn. It
would be good. It would be over in two hours.

10

———— ·•· ————

Stuck in the Valley

The soup is not my best. It's too strong with too much garlic. The healing agents won't help if she pukes. I dilute by half again with water. That's better, but she'll still complain, which means she won't eat it. Still, it's better than what they're serving, so I get the soup into the Thermos, and the journey continues.

Where does the time go? It's dark again and windy with slanting rain, but it's not yet seven so I can enter through the ER, through the smoking section on the corner, where the street people patients hang out in hospital jammies, tethered intravenously. They hearken to my arrival, some for the smell of soup but most to see if I'm a smoker who might spare a few. Wouldn't you just know it; I'm flush with spare change but have no smokes.

Inside, down the hall and around the corner I enter the elevator and rise. On the third floor two no-nonsense nurses, women in XL, come on with a multi-tiered cart holding hundreds of small trays, each with a combo of pills, tablets, syringe(s), compresses, elixirs, tonics, suppositories, depressants, mood elevators, salves, unguents and ointments. They chide me for helping the cart clear the elevator door. "Don't touch that! Stand there. There. Hands down, please. Don't touch."

I don't think contamination is an issue, because the cart looks less than sterile. Maybe they think I want their drugs. I don't, so I smile. They glare, like I'm interfering. So I ask, "Why are you so glum? The pre-op guys were cutting up like a cocktail party? They have all the fun."

They exit on seven. At nine I exit and walk down to the west wing to find that we've given up our private room to a little boy who fell and banged his head and isn't doing well. She's the last adult on the ward, so maybe things are easing up in the neurology wing.

The new space is a share, curtained off from a bigger space, though the curtain is five feet short of closing. Another patient nearby may be a woman. In the four hundred pound range, she's splayed like a frog on a dissection board. Tubes, hoses, spikes, pressure lines, clamps, braces and flex drains confine her. All fluids flush continuously into a main canal. She can move only her vocal cords and bowels. Her waste sump is another flow that joins the flow from her lungs, through a scupper over the main canal. I can't believe she's alive, and I can't look with ease, but the array is too rare to turn away from. The lungs are exposed. Fluids flow. She makes sounds and movements indicating the end, perhaps seeking it.

Rachel told the cancer survivors, *You're all doing the right thing.* I tell the unfortunate woman, "You're doing the right thing." She doesn't respond.

The new nurse is Nate, a bright-eyed, friendly fellow. Rachel seems calm, so I take him for a good nurse, but then I see that Rachel is not so much calm as frozen. I walk around to the far side and see the problem. Her face and neck on that side are bruised and mushy as an overripe melon. The eye is swollen shut. She looks as battered as George Foreman in the fourteenth and just as tired.

The check valve and turkey baster removed earlier from the base of the skull are back in place. Why? So the fluid causing this swelling can dissipate. That should occur in only ten more hours, or maybe twelve.

The swelling isn't necessarily the result of the angiogram, but we can't be certain. In any event, the final invasiveness is done, the baseline secure.

Also present is Claudia, the charge nurse. Claudia wears granny glasses, a crewcut and a stern face. She's smaller than me but won't look up. "It sounds soothing," I say. Nate and Claudia turn my way. "Like a Zen fountain." I mean the layered flushing three steps over. I harken to it, and Nate laughs short.

Claudia finishes her adjustments and walk out as the splayed patient nearby wails, "Ohhh . . . Whoah . . . Oohh." Nurse Claudia and Nurse Nate confer in the hall and then leave.

"My God," Rachel says. I wonder where the Zen-fountain woman's family is and who is allowing this application of the healing arts. I set my things down and announce chicken soup, my best yet. Rachel joins the moaning chorus. I assure her that eating this soup is not required. But sooner or later, eat she must. She says she can't. She keeps her hand on her spherical face as if to realize it, maybe monitoring for deflation.

"Fine. Don't eat. I'll put some clear broth in a cup. If you don't like it, we'll throw it out." I hand her the cup.

She sips and says, "It's delicious. I can't eat." She sets it aside. I sit. We stare. Rachel drifts in and out of sleep. The wailing is chaotic and painful, without rhythm. The beeps and buzzes up and down the ICU are syncopated. The system is automatic, so that a critical margin in any vital function of any patient on the corridor will override all other monitors on the corridor. So anyone approaching the big D will trigger the alarm on all monitors with concurrent flashing of the room number and vital function(s) of the patient on the brink at the moment. So I don't need to panic every time our monitor goes off like a nickel slot jackpot. It's a child down the way in trouble. I wonder what happens when several kids trigger alarms at once. I'm told it gets insane on the ward, and I'm again amazed at the dedication required for a single shift, yet this level of activity seems addictive—or maybe personal satisfaction keeps them going. It's an adrenaline rush at any rate, along with fundamental goodness in most of them.

An alarm sounds on the monitor, and I look up to see that it's us. Not to worry—a plastic crinkle follows the intermittent flashing, and I relax as another bag of Gatorade occludes. Nate is there with a full bag. He moves deftly and appears to be happy with his work. So I ask how we're doing. "Are you kidding?" he says. "She's conscious. She's talking. She has no apparent limitations. She's off the charts."

Off the charts. I suppose the Zen-fountain woman is at the base of the bell curve. Nate is cooking something up. I ask what he's doing. "Oh, this. We're changing—. Well. We're changing the . . . Oh. Well . . . Well, heck, I guess it's okay to tell you this . . ."

I guess it's okay to tell you this? Whatever it is, I'd like to know what's not okay to tell us. Why is secrecy so integral to the system? Of course some risks are calculated, and an educated team with data to drawn on will presumably choose best. It's a difficult moment, realizing that these scenes may be revisited in court. "You guess it's okay? What could possibly not be okay to tell us?"

"I mean, it was written up in the New England Journal of Medicine. We're changing her anti-seizure medication. The Dilantin is attacking her white blood cells. Her count is dangerously low."

"What?" I react in a personal way. He's a good nurse—at least he tells the truth. But ignorance is not best for us, and our two cents should be worth more than that. Still, the assessment/advise and consent format will not factor our opinions, as if that exclusion is necessary to serve in a timely manner. That exclusion is also the likely cause of tension, redundancy and error, given the staff assigned to profile patients and psychiatric needs.

"Yeah. It happens. We're going to put her on Valporic Acid. It'll prevent the seizures without taking her white blood count so low."

"You said dangerously low."

He shrugs, tight-lipped, afraid to go further. I think he's only as good as the system allows, and the honesty of the system is compromised. "How will this change in medication show up on the chart?"

He shrugs again. "Here. See? It says the time and Valporic Acid and the dosage?"

"But I see no reference or any mention of dangerously reduced white blood cells. Or any reference to Dilantin as a source of danger. And why didn't we use Valporic Acid in the first place?" I scan the chart in reverse, from now to yesterday. It logs each dose of Dilantin right up to the first dose of Valporic Acid but never mentions fewer white blood cells. Could the system be so sinister in its self-defense, to the point of cover-up? Is this a symptom of systemic paranoia?

"Can you believe that?" Rachel groans. The process feels experimental. Nate assures us that nobody wants a lowered white blood count, but seizure is a very real threat now, and Dilantin gives the most clinically significant results historically.

"We're experimenting here?" He doesn't know the answer to that, which may be defensible. "Go, Nate. Make your rounds." He smiles and complies. Yes, we are a pain in the tuchas, but a moment of inclusion could have kept me busy, calling around to find a less risky remedy for seizure prevention.

We sit. We stare. We wait. Nurse Janet arrives with a serving tray of unguents, orange ointment mostly, which she sets aside during examination of the wound. "Oh, my," she says, her happy face in mild alarm.

"What?" we ask on cue.

"Whoever did these sutures really laced you up right. It's so flat and tight. I think you're fine."

"What are you looking for?" I ask.

"Leaks," she says casually.

Rachel's good eye opens wide. "My brains are going to leak out?"

"Oh, ho, ho, ho ... No, ho, ho," Nurse Janet assures. "But they could! We had to cut the seal. You know the brain has a waterproof seal all the way around it, and we had to cut yours open, you know."

"So now she could leak?" I ask.

"Oh, yes. Until you heal."

"You mean the seal restores itself to waterproof?"

Nurse Janet nods. "It takes about a year."

Rachel asks, "So stuff could leak in too?"

"No, ho, ho."

"What if I'm snorkeling and I dive down and hit my head on a rock."

"Oh, my," Nurse Janet says. "To tell you the truth, I don't know if I would snorkel anymore, if I were you."

Rachel and I turn to Nurse Janet in disbelief. Nurse Janet responds as a friend in confidence. "You know this could happen again at any time, driving down the road, in an airplane. On an elevator. Snorkeling—Oh, my."

"What difference does it make?" Rachel asks. "It could happen right now, right here, talking to you in this God-forsaken room." Nurse Janet droops in resignation to our woeful outlook. She pats Rachel's head, as if to commiserate. Rachel looks away. "I'd rather be under water with friends."

"Now, now."

"Are you done?" I ask. She is, and like a good listener if not a good conciliator, she leaves. We sit. On the overhead TV Hollywooders in tuxedos and fabulous gowns present each other with prizes for excellence. We don't listen because the sound would be tedious, and anyway, the lips are easy to read. Many thanks for making this possible and all those who helped, without whom we could not blah, blah, blah. I think we're getting old; we recognize so few of the newly fabulous.

Sue arrives. Rachel brightens, anxious to share. "Look what they've done! Look at my face!"

To Sue's credit, she shrugs it off. "Oh, I know! But you're doing so well!"

"This place is so . . ." In three seconds Rachel's heart rate on the monitor goes from sixty-five to ninety. I call Sue outside abruptly and explain the need for calmness. I ask that she please keep an eye on the monitor to know how Rachel is doing. Sue understands, but back at the gurney the sisters wind up again, waving their hands and racing their hearts. Sue brought hats and scarves, and now they try them on over the gore and stitching, roughing up the works. I ask, please, for calmness. I am told to go, have some fun. So I go to another ninth floor, which is my office a mile away, where I drink many beers and fall asleep on the sofa.

Sunday and Monday pass slowly, mostly sitting, watching the overhead TV, standing guard, listening to nonstop dings and alarms and the endless lament of the Zen-fountain woman. I take breaks, walk down-town and back up the hill. I stretch and breathe deep and wonder what I'd be doing if this had gone the other way. I'd sell the house. I'd move, I think. I don't know where. I'd find homes for . . . well, Clarisse, I think; she's so new and would make a good pet with proper care. Ed and Stella could stay together, but Dewey and Flojo . . . I couldn't . . . Nor with Molly and Dino. I'd . . . Never mind. It didn't go that way. I take Elmer Fudd's car back and get my car. I make calls to family and friends.

Rachel eats only yogurt and juice, refusing further bulk until she's allowed to get up and move. Sue comes daily with the scrabble board. They play. Rachel wins. I would suspect Sue let her win, but they've played for years and take it personally.

A woman named Nancy visits daily with an array of electronic gadgetry, including amplifiers and sensors. She reads the flow and pressure in the vessels of each square centimeter of the brain. Then she marks the chart. This is Doppler Ultrasound. The final rating is a function of multiple denominators over the cosine of the logarithm divided by the discount and surcharge or something or other. A final rating of thirty and above indicates vasospasm, a constriction of blood vessels indicating the onset of a stroke. Rachel rates 29.3, which is technically below the line, but it's too close for discharge from the ICU, where stroke potential is best monitored and urgent procedures best implemented in the event of a stroke.

We're marginally comforted by constant assurance that *everyone* has *some* vasospasm and a convulsion or two may be normal in this tender phase. Rachel wants to know what this daily Doppler Ultrasound proce-dure is going to cost, because to her it's bells and whistles, and she is still able to tell if she's not feeling well, all by herself. I tell her the insurance will cover, but she insists that a rip is a rip. Nurse Nancy tells her it's only four hundred dollars per test, and she proceeds with another test.

Monday is a milestone; the dipstick comes out of her skull. The steel spike screwed through her head to monitor brain pressure is no longer necessary because we're beyond the critical risk time for brain swelling. Dipstick removal is a tangible relief but comes with searing pain. "How much pain?" Nurse Amy wants to know.

"How much pain? It hurts," Rachel says.

"On a one to ten scale, one being the mildest, and ten being the worst."

"Five," Rachel says. Nurse Amy enters five on the computer and dispenses Tylenol.

Worse yet, when Rachel tilts her head from dead level, yellow goo spills out. This is demoralizing.

But the shift soon changes and Nurse Leah is back, which is a great thing, because she's the best of the staff on comfort and mechanical assistance. She makes us wonder about the education and job-interview process. Surely compassion cannot be taught, but it could be reviewed with a few pointers. Leah dabs the hole and sets a piece of gauze on top and restates the staff shibboleth: "This is normal." Her touch is soft, her demeanor warm and reassuring, until the next arrival.

Nurse Claudia, the angry woman with the crewcut and granny glasses who runs the floor this shift, announces that the hospital is full. Rachel no longer qualifies for intensive care and would be moved now, but with no vacancy on three, she must wait till tomorrow. Rachel has hovered less than a point below the line for three days, but in view of her impressive progress, Nurse Claudia is willing to forego the critical risk period for vasospasm, seven days. They warned us of seven-day risk, but in view of our unique recovery potential, I'm grateful for the shift in policy. I concur with Claudia.

"Jesus, I want to go home. I'll never get out of here," Rachel moans.

"Oh, the third floor feels like a hotel with room service after this," Leah says, stepping forward. "You can close the door down on the third floor. No noise." We ponder no noise, briefly. Nurse Claudia reminds us that early departure from intensive care can only occur after a favorable reading on the Doppler Ultrasound measuring flow and pressure in Rachel's cranial blood vessels.

"Boy oh boy," Rachel mutters, counting the coupons she had to clip to save the four hundred dollars spent on one day's testing. But she smiles; parole looks possible. Tuesday should be the big day. If the machine needs another few hun, so be it. We want out.

But it's not to be. I take Tuesday morning to stretch again on a long walk down to Rainier Square for new underwear and a new shirt and return to gloom. Doppler Ultrasound Nancy did it wrong, Rachel says, blowing our chance for freedom. Rachel is distraught among the beeps and dings and flashing lights. The Zen-fountain woman wails and groans, and Rachel seems oddly aligned with the chorus. She hasn't slept fifty minutes in a row now for seven days.

"What do you mean, she did it wrong?"

"She pulled my neck. It's still killing me. And she took the reading right when Sue was here, and we . . . I . . ." She can't speak. Tears well up.

"You were excited?" She nods, crying now. "You think that changed your reading?" She nods again. Now she sobs; Sue was winning, but then Rachel saw an opening for a triple-score multiple word play in a tight corner that would give her the game—a thirty-six-pointer! She got excited and now thinks the machine read her wrong. Besides that, the ultrasound woman pulled her head so far to the side that it ripped the sutures from the gang valve in the jugular vein. This occurred, Rachel says, because the woman didn't want to move the machinery cart around to the other side of the bed, where the reading should be taken.

For the first time she's openly crying, practically in harmony with the Zen-fountain woman. The difference between the two is that Rachel always took care of herself as well as those around her. Yet here she is, feeling trapped, devoid of autonomous care and no better off than an obese geriatric or a perfectly good dog waiting to go home. She regrets again that she consented to surgery. She doesn't mind dying, she says; she wants to die. She wants out of this horrible, horrible place.

Of course she's whining, feeling the effects of sleep deprivation, mild starvation and endless trespass on her body, inside and out. Worst of all, she can't stand her hair, shaved off in a minute, and now it won't grow back for years. Her head is covered with crusty yellow snot, and it itches. She hasn't washed in five days, and her skin hurts from lying down for seven days, and she can't sleep more than two winks without some cheerful attendant waking her up for a triviality. I can't stand to see her cry, especially now, having weathered the worst with courage, only to falter on the small stuff. But I sense fundamental weakening from the core again, from the source of her relentless happiness. She is not happy. She is sad. Along with that comes an ashen color suggesting death.

The bells ring, the buzzers buzz. It's like Vegas. We can't go home, and we're crapping out. Children up and down the ward pre-empt each other with more daring proximity to death. Alarms transcend final buzzers, and the Zen-fountain woman drowns them all with, "Oooohhh! Whaoa! Oaooooh!" Rachel places a hand on her left temporal lobe. It hurts.

I tell her I'll be right back. I don't know if she can hear me or if she cares any longer what I have to say. But I can't help seeking usefulness. I think depression can resolve independently more easily than with a significant other constantly shooing it away. I find Nurse Leah and briefly relate the headache and the onset of depression and its possible cure. She takes me at face value, perhaps the only person here to do so. Rachel is not her patient today, she says, but she'll see that hair washing is scheduled. If it's not done by the end of the shift, she'll stay and do it.

I go back to the binging bonging flashing space and tell Rachel that her hair will be washed. She wants to know when. I tell her it could happen any time but it may not happen till the shift change. That could be twelve hours, she says, weeping hopelessly as a child suffering a loss in the family.

The open space where the curtain once hung is now filled with Nurse Jane, the stridently happy one who looked for leaks. Jane's happiness seems rote and practiced; she doesn't know us but says she's seen it many times. She sounds like day-in, day-out with another testimonial to lowest common denominators. Nurse Jane assures us that she knows what we're feeling, what we felt and what we'll feel next. She means well but doesn't know squat about us.

"Now, now," she offers. "You'll be out of here in no time." Her deep, grating voice is that of a sternly loving mother to a deeply saddened child.

We wait to see why she's here, crowding our little space. She bats her lashes and asks, "Do you have a headache?" Do we ever. I tell her Rachel's is five point five four. Mine is a solid eight. Can you help? She complies, recording vital data for Rachel, telling me not to worry, that nobody will miss these two Tylenol; they'll be just our little secret.

She perks up, as if this interlude between depression and Tylenol is a perfect opening for counseling. It's not, but she proceeds: "Do you have children?" She's all smiles and sparkle now on the subject that all people love. Ah, children; that's the ticket. Because if you remind people they're doing something for the children, they'll stop bawling and be happy, thinking of the children. "Yes," I say. "We have seven."

"Seven! Oh, my!" She beams joyfully. "Seven children!" Eight would be better and would make us appear more rational. Rachel gives me the dirty look but has no strength to back it up. "How old is the youngest?" Nurse Jane is quite engaged now.

"Not even a year," I say. "Stella is what? Ten months?" Nurse Jane stops in mid-beam to eyeball our chart. She's taken aback, perhaps considering an addition of DELUSIONAL to PARANOID. I'm past the big five oh. Rachel is forty-seven. We are not so far removed from procreative viability, and for only a few hundred grand and the resources available here, we could have a litter.

But Nurse Jane smells a bullshitter in the woodpile. Over a fragmenting gush she realizes that this warm and fuzzy chitchat is with two nutcases who think they had a child ten months ago. Rachel pulls my plug. "We have five cats and two dogs. We have no children."

"Oh!" Nurse Jane titters. "Five cats and two dogs! Weh, heh, hell, I'm sure they're just like children to you!"

I want to challenge Nurse Jane's and the team's presumption on rationale and the perception of paranoia relative to stability. *We're all under pressure here* feels more like a credo defining a value system, in which many children and the miracle available here are rational and best. We are apparently peas of a very different pod. Nurse Jane is here for sympathy and understanding, but she's not of our context. Well intentioned, to be sure, she is presumptuous and not applicable.

But I too am all used up. So I go along with a little laugh: got you, Jane. Good one, huh? Jane titters, and I suggest, "If you wouldn't mind, Nurse Jane, Rachel needs her hair washed in thirty minutes. Between now and then could you please see that we're not interrupted by anyone?"

"I'd love to help you wash your hair but I have three other patients, and that's thirty minutes out of my day, so I don't think that can happen."

"How many patients does Leah have?"

"Three. She was supposed to be your nurse but we switched because the little guy she was working with yesterday really wanted her."

"I wonder why."

"I'll try to help if I can. I just . . ."

"That's fine. Could we have some privacy?" She leaves. Another nurse enters. I admonish politely as I can, but it still comes out, "Get out, please." It's been seven days, nonstop. This nurse also leaves, pulling the curtain behind her.

I give it a minute to calm down but doubt that this space is ever calm, which is counterintuitive to healing. The place rotates like a tube of broken glass with no mirror to reflect symmetry and no beauty. Nothing thrives here; you only get more breakage, chaotic refraction and sharp edges.

Rachel is inconsolable. It's seven days now of no solid food, no physical movement and no sound sleep, except of course for the anesthesia during brain surgery. What a nap.

"We're going to change our strategy," I say.

"We don't have a strategy. We gave up. Unless maybe we had a secret plan that I'd sneak up on them and jump in bed and make them slice me up and poke me full of nails."

I laugh. "That's very good. You are doing terrific. Now we're going to get out of here."

"Oh, right."

"We need calmness. Inner calmness. We can change your pressure and flow. I know we can."

"I'm going to die," she says.

"That's okay," I say. "Go ahead. Die in your mind anyway."

"Great. Should I close my eyes?"

"Yes. Listen: Do you remember when we dabbled in meditation?"

Of course she must. It was only a few years ago during the breast cancer resolution. She didn't really respond to my suggestion of meditation, but when the healers and other non-surgical counselors called for visualization, she wanted to try it—not meditation but visualization. I explained to her that there is no difference between the two, that visualization is meditation with imagery. Imagery is an integral component of internal change. And death is a primary image.

She lay listless, tears rolling, eyes closed.

"Do you remember what I told you? With death comes new life. You've done this. I have to tell you, I think it's an extremely small number of people who have the chance of doing that, you know, dying in your mind, and now you get to do it twice."

"Oh, boy," she squeaks over the knot in her throat.

"Die in your mind as if everything before is over. Then we begin. Imagine a body of water, deep and still. Imagine it from now on, at least until this time tomorrow. You can keep your eyes closed or open. It doesn't matter. But as much as you can, imagine water, deep and still."

We share the watery imagery, until she opens her eyes and says, "I have to pee."

By now she's adept at unplugging herself. The intravenous leads are easily snapped apart at fittings in the lines near the injectors. She sits up and pulls them all off. I unplug the monitor, stow the cord and help wheel her to the potty seat. We get her back into the bed and re-plugged. "Sometime tonight you'll have your hair washed and you'll be cleaned. No more scrabble between now and tomorrow. No more visits. Talk between us will be minimal. We'll meditate our way out of here."

"Yes. And in a little while you'll walk out of here. You'll have a beer and breathe some air. You'll be able to sleep."

"Please." She sighs and closes her eyes.

We sustain silence, or at least what can be salvaged of it for an hour, till she opens her eyes and says, "Please go." She is on the verge of tears again, her face half swollen and drawn deep in sadness. I can't help but mirror her feeling, for we do suffer a death in the family, one that meditation cannot assuage. I press on for calmness. I rise slowly and move to her. I bend and kiss her and tell her we're on our way out of here. I promise to get her out of here by tomorrow, if she'll only go along with my little game.

She neither speaks nor nods. I tell her I love her more than ever. She grimaces, as if such words are patronization at this point. Look at her, all carved up with a shaved head and fifty-six stitches where silky blonde hair used to be. Two dozen sensors and needles stick out of her arms and legs. A few more are pasted all over her chest. Her skin is sallow and drawn. One eye is swollen shut and seeping. The other is dark and baggy.

"No shit. I couldn't do this like you. Not that you're doing it as well as you did yesterday. But you did it. You're doing it. You're a major player. Off the charts. I didn't doubt that you could do it, but you're standing pretty tall right now. I can't believe how rare you are, to get to do this twice." She smiles uncertainly for an opportunity she surely could have lived happily without. I put my hands on her chest, on her shoulders, on her cheeks.

I leave.

Nurse Jane watches from the corridor, waiting with more sympathy and misunderstanding. I attempt a smile and say, "She's always been happy to a fault. Exceedingly happy. This depression worries me, and I know you're busy. But I can tell you she's inherently happy because her needs are so simple. You may think that a woman like her asking to have her hair washed is casual or vain or—"

"No, I don't think that at all. I just don't know if I'll have time."

"All I'm saying is that she's severely depressed, and a hair wash could go a long way in cheering her up. Maybe if you viewed it as a mood elevating drug or a minor procedure. You know she hasn't slept or eaten or moved around in eight days now. This place is taking a toll. She's still at critical risk for spasm and seizure, and I think if washing her hair could lift her spirits, then maybe it should be a priority."

Nurse Jane wants to comfort me but only in the confines of her understanding. She takes initiative now, sharing her true feelings with a tough customer, one who could perhaps benefit from the insight and experience of the staff here. "You know," she begins. "This was unavoidable. This depression. I think it's for the best. My professional opinion is that it's a necessary part of acceptance. She's only now finally hearing what we've been trying to tell you, that—"

"No, Jane. You still don't get it." I smile to compensate my own understanding. "Rachel heard you and all the staff the first time, but you have yet to hear her. You're worse than Christians around here, with your God-awful righteousness and rightness. Anyone who doesn't agree with you or go along with your understanding is irrational. We come from a different belief system, Jane. We wouldn't be here if we had a choice, but we don't have a choice, so we're going along with your religion as far as we can. But you should make no more mistakes, and please, no more presumptions. She has no reason to be depressed other than this overwhelmingly depressing place. Will you please make time to help her wash her hair?"

I am in Nurse Jane's face, so to speak. This, too, Jane understands, but to what advantage or with what reception I cannot tell. She nods, nearly tearful herself, which may be cause for hope. She promises to wash Rachel's hair if she can find the time. I assure her I can ask for no more than her best effort.

Nurse Jane and I go our separate ways on that fragile truce. I descend and depart and drive ten blocks to where I sit and stare, till I tire and walk to the sofa where I lie down and sleep.

I rise early and call. I am patched through, and Rachel says, "Good morning, dear. I got my hair washed. I feel much better. I'm going to—"

"Sh . . . Water. Deep and still."

"Oh. Yeah. Okay. Are you coming down?"

"Soon."

11

———◆———

Free at Last

Iarrive at eight. We sit in repose until ten-thirty, when a man comes to fix the sound on the TV. I didn't know it was broken. Rachel says that it can't go up loud enough to drown the wailing of the Zen-fountain woman, but it helps.

At eleven the Doppler Ultrasound woman arrives. We're watching the science fiction network, where a woman is being interviewed on her ability to channel another soul, whose voice comes through her body much differently than her own voice. The other voice says things the channel woman would never know to say. How could she?

The Doppler Ultrasound woman is still Nancy. She is methodical and formal, saying she'll need a few minutes to get set up. The TV is a drain on meditative repose in the normal world, but here it helps homogenize the ambient chaos.

Following the woman who channels another soul is a practicing psychiatrist, on hand to explain the channeling phenomenon. He says the woman creates a belief in her subconscious mind that this event is actually happening, so she's legitimate instead of fraudulent.

"She believes, you see," the shrink says. "That's how we differentiate between legitimacy and fraud. But that's all it is, a personal belief. It's not really happening."

"I could have told you that," Nancy says, tweaking her diodes and capacitors, prepping the goo that goes on the skin to facilitate the ultrasound test. We turn off the TV to dwell on the still waters at hand.

By way of transition, I tell Nancy, "You express your personal beliefs, Nancy. But how can you know your personal beliefs are sounder than that woman's beliefs? What makes you believe you're right in your beliefs?" Nancy doesn't need this. She only wants to clear another test, moving onward to sundown and payday. "Belief is personal by nature, Nancy. Let me give you an example."

She waits tolerantly, but when I take my place at the foot of the bed, sitting on the edge of a chair with good posture, chest open, hands on knees, eyes mostly closed, body still, she doesn't press. She proceeds.

Anyone in proximity to Doppler Ultrasound can attest to its uniquely eerie sound. Maybe we set the stage for it, dousing the TV and our own talk, going snake-eyed with good posture or as close to it as we can manage, conjuring imagery of slow flow and calm waters. The room quickly fills with the Doppler Ultrasound of stellar bodies in their hurtle through space—they and the attending spirits are with us at full speed, right there in 909 West. We feel no friction because you have none in space, and we scream across the cosmos. We hurl so fast along with the spirits, both good spirits and bad, light spirits and dark, that we needn't sort them out. We are all of all at full speed. We move fast but slow, seeking only calmness in the whirl, peace at the speed of light.

After sounding the vessels on each square centimeter over the left temporal lobe and adjacent area, Nancy sets a hand on Rachel's forehead to pull it her way, so she can get readings from the other side of the head, the far side. But she stops when I stop her, speaking gently: "No, Nancy. We'll have no head pulling today. And no neck twisting. Move your machine to the other side of the bed."

Nancy doesn't need this either, and since it represents real effort, she glances up, prelude to a what-for. But if sweet looks could kill she'd be dead. She smiles back at me, neither sweetly nor sincerely and certainly not more than halfway. She moves the whole shebang to the other side of the bed, grunting and groaning, less methodically and formally and with a great show of effort.

Rachel retains her repose, and in no time the spirits can be heard soaring and looping and whooshing about the room again.

In a few minutes we're done. Nancy scans the printout, nods slowly and wrinkles her forehead. "These are better. Much better," she says.

"How can you tell? You haven't worked the formula."

"Oh, you can tell when you've done this as long as I have."

"I hope you're right, Nancy. I hope you can tell what happened here, too." She laughs short. "I don't like to think that you're close-minded here. But I do wish you could open up to things beyond the dogma. You might consider possibilities. Like that woman on TV and what she believes is happening every time you believe something else is happening. You might consider the difference between explaining something and explaining something away. That's a pitfall for people who work here too long. You feel compelled to explain everything else away."

She is curt on her departure. Rachel is relieved that it's done and we have apparently passed. She is up, disconnecting, unplugging and packing her things. I remind her that the place runs like molasses, that she should retain her meditative repose. She asks what for. I laugh and tell her: for no reason at all.

In a while Sue arrives with a new game, cribbage, because scrabble is suspect.

I take my leave to get lunch and begin reentry to the world of livelihood. I think this vacation could be the most expensive yet.

The end. Or the beginning of the next phase at any rate. Who can tell when it's actually over, short of gasping and realizing what your last thought will actually be? The highs and lows don't stop. Like the night of the day of liberation from intensive care.

I return at seven to find that Rachel is officially released but still waits in the maelstrom. Pam is the new nurse and is very busy with patients in greater need of service. I'm glad she's scarce, but we need to push that last official documentation that will allow this inertia to break.

Pam tells me that I must learn to be patient sooner or later and now is as good a time as any, so why don't I sit down and behave for a change? We haven't met, so I know I'm suspect on the ward. Never mind. Pam must make a call and sign off so Rachel can move to the third floor, but she blocks like a defensive linewoman. She too is suspect, proving a point.

I find Nurse Claudia, who is again the charge nurse and has also had enough of an overbearing, reflexive resister like me. She admonishes, "They know she's coming down. We spoke to them. They said they'll come and get us when they're ready, and that's what they'll do. They have patients to discharge down there, and until they do, they have no room for your wife."

"What time was that?"

"Listen, Mister. This is a hospital. A trauma center. Nobody cares about your personal comfort. We have emergencies all the time here, so things get pushed back. Now, go on down there and have a seat or get out."

I don't doubt her sincerity, but here too common sense preempts her impatience. "Are you going to tell me what time that was? Or do I have to ask on the third floor?"

"It was three o'clock."

"Does this hospital actually discharge people at eight o'clock at night?"

"No. We don't."

"Then a room is either waiting right now on the third floor, or it's not. That means either you will call them right now, or I'll go down there. If the room is ready, I'll take my wife down there. If it's not, we'll go home. It's on you."

Boy, does she ever hate a pushy jerk like me, one who is better off neutralized with a phone call than set up for more macho noise. But she's not going to make the call with me standing there, so I can just go on down there and have a seat.

She makes the call but doesn't like it. I wait around the corner. It's rhubarb, rhubarb, mumbo jumbo, till she heats up on a gasp of disbelief. She nearly chokes, "What? No! *You* were going to call *us*! Since three? Well, that's just great! This asshole is reading me the riot act, and I'm telling him to get the hell out of here. That's just great!"

I'm waiting when she rounds the corner. I preempt her again with, "We'll be getting ready. In ten minutes we're heading down, with or without a field guide."

The field guide arrives five minutes later, a much larger woman who may not be a candidate for a relationship with Nurse Claudia but only because the larger woman is much happier. She freely concedes that this system will work you stupid unless you work it first. She rambles, "You would not believe how many people would have sat there all damn night waiting for something to fix itself out of thin air. I'll tell you something else; that room there in Intensive? That room runs you two thousand dollars a day. You're sitting there at midnight: Bingo! Two grand, baby."

The world changes in an elevator ride. We're rolled to a room with four walls, a door and a bathroom with a shower. The window overlooks Elliott Bay, and the door closes to blessed silence, but not before Rachel springs off the gurney so fast her gown flies open, exposing her back end. "Oh, I'm liking this!" the big nurse says.

"Oh, yeah, she's resilient," I say, and the big nurse squints at me, like I'm blind to the Promised Land.

In mere minutes we're alone again, back among the living silence. Rachel is happy again, grinning and knowing she's on her way. I go down to the car and bring up the dozen bouquets that arrived in the last few days. No flowers are allowed in Intensive Care. They're wilting now yet glorious in effusion of color and scent.

The next morning I'm jolted awake by a phone call at seven. But it's okay—the attending physician came around and asked why she's still in the hospital. She is discharged. The paper shuffle will take two hours. She'll be done by nine. With another shot of adrenaline that I know is inching me nearer the big one, I lunge to pee, shower, dress and drive down. She's dressed and packed when I get there, and I weaken on seeing her with a silk scarf tied around her head like Aunt Jemima used to wear. She's radiant again, again happy and ready to ride.

Speet Patorogy comes around to assure us we're doing all right. Physical rehab says it will be dicey the next few days. I tell this nurse she's in denial; Rachel could click her heels and win a race around the block.

The pharmacist is downstairs waiting with a grocery bag—a big brown paper one, no shit—full of drugs. In a minute we're in the car and in five we're in the office, because maybe it's better that we spend the night in town rather than ninety minutes away.

Rachel nearly swoons with excitement at proximity to familiar objects like a desk and rugs and a computer and a couch and windows that open to fresh air and a locked door and perfect privacy. She raises her arms and grins. Then she lies down just for a bit, for a four-hour nap.

She wants to be held now and again, to claim her place among the living.

It's been twenty years, but the next two months were another adventure. Nothing brought her back up more than homecoming with the dogs and cats, and the thousand flowers crowding the garden, blossoming in celebration. She stood before a tulip cluster thick with baby's breath. She opened her arms in salutation to life.

We did not return to routine, nor was she physically whole for a year or two. But then neither am I. Those first days passed like life anew, in happy surrender. We stretched and walked and ate well. The days took what they required and returned an intangible that I think of as light. Rachel strapped on the harnesses in the kitchen and the yard. She knew she couldn't handle the wheelbarrow if it was completely loaded. Nor could she shovel, unless it was only mulch. What could mulch weigh? We had our ups and downs on what must not be done. I think she remained in denial for a while on her close encounter with death. She accused me frequently and unjustly of overbearing demeanor and judgmental disposition. She resented my accusation of drunkenness when she had in fact sustained a massive cerebral hemorrhage. Processing the event allowed her to sit still, so we sat and talked it over.

I didn't mind her accusation. I asked: if you take the judge from judgmental, what's left but the mental? And what's wrong with seeing the difference between right and wrong? Isn't personal perception part of instinct and intuition and therefore prerequisite to rational behavior? Besides, I don't judge anyone but people.

What you get, she said, is a nice man who knows how to keep his mouth shut. She was wrong, but I loved the repartee. Nor did I care if she used wrong words sometimes. I still can't tell if the frequency of misuse is diminishing. For a long time she said her CDs when she meant CAT scans. She might have called the lawn mower the vacuum cleaner or referred to her brain as her motor. She said they put the Titanic in her head, meaning titanium. Then again it could have been the Titanic. She told her friends it didn't matter at all. She meant that the titanium didn't matter relative to airport security. People didn't know that's what she meant, but that didn't matter either.

Her denial faded slowly, I think, making room for the awful realization of what an outing in town for a few beers turned into. She read aloud to me from the hundred pages she pulled down from the Internet. Given time and breathing room and distance from the war zone and the nonstop assault, she could accept and believe what she resisted so stridently. "Listen to this," she said. "'One third of people with ruptured aneurysms die before they get to the hospital. One third die after they get to the hospital. Of the remaining third, forty percent end up with neurological problems that make life difficult.'" These stats were taken from www.brain-surgery.com/aneurysm.html.

I reminded Rachel that young Dr. Michael, the frail fellow who first examined her, gave us these stats as part of his presentation. She insisted he did not, but she concedes large gaps in her memory of those few days, so maybe he did. She knows he did not give her the average on post-op hospital time for this condition. The average post-op stay is three more weeks in intensive care followed by two more weeks in a regular room. If he had, she would never have gone along.

As it was, she was back on the street six days after surgery, which makes the statistics suspect, possibly polluted with the dire bad habits of a slovenly society. If you eat burgers and get no exercise and take pharmaceutical drugs for whatever ails you and carry too much fat, then the statistics are yours to bear. Avoid those things, and the stats are usually beaten.

Moreover, she stared off in thought more often, as if realizing at last the long odds against a full recovery. She doesn't drool or limp. She's still a dynamic chef who would rather play around in the kitchen than cruise a mall. She still turns heads in a classy dress, maybe mine most of all, and she's still back at work in the shipping department.

Her shaved head grew out an inch in the first two months. She still flopped hair from the other side like a bald guy in denial, but it worked much better on her. She rolled the scarf like a headband and wore it over the top, tying it off behind her neck. And she grinned, taking it off for those who wanted to see, perversely balancing her self-consciousness with zero inhibition.

We lost ourselves in motorcycling for many more miles after that, and she could still hang on with the best of them.

On the first the anniversary of our marriage after the aneurism, I give her a pendant, an aquamarine surrounded by diamonds. She was taken aback with the extravagance and blushed, saying she had no place to wear it. I told her that the pendant was in gratitude for a lasting lesson in imagery and strength; that sooner or later everyone wakes up dog-butt ugly, and she took her turn with Olympian spirit. But she no longer fears the loss of physical beauty, reminding me of her strength.

"I don't know if everyone sooner or later shines," I said. She thought I'd begun my usual sentimental pap, but I'd thought things over. I advised her that the aquamarine charm was not for her. It was a gift from her and me to the angels who were all over her one night only a few weeks prior and still are. I assured her of this reality. "I saw it here, just over your face, with my own eyes. This charm says thank you. You wear it in the garden or shagging stray cats or thumping melons, squeezing tomatoes or splitting firewood or packing snorkel gear—wherever you go. You wear it for them."

She asked if I thought she would die of cancer or aneurysm. I told her I thought she would go quietly of old age. She said she couldn't be so sure of that, and given a choice, at least aneurysm is quick. I conceded that her swan song may be quick, but I thought it would be decades away, in her sleep. "You sense phantoms around every corner once you've been mugged," I said. "Give it a few years, you'll be your old, cocky self."

"No, I don't," she corrected me. "I don't sense bad things. I never did." She taught me that widows and widowers might think they know what a gone spouse would think or say or feel. But they don't know. She confided that she no longer saw things in her peripheral vision like she did, but something was present. She saw it mostly in the old part of the house, the original part built in 1927 that has held generations of people in their best pursuits, cooking, eating and talking. I asked if this presence felt ominous, and she says it did not. She thought in fact that we were welcome there, that these things, if they were things, may have played a part on the day of her hemorrhage.

"You think that was a good day?"

"Well, sure it was good. It was for the best. They let me know my brain thingie was, you know, in there. Oh, I think it was all for the best." What a nut. Yet she reminded me of my affront to society, peeing on the floor at Home Improvement World, a behavior not yet resolved. I shrugged, indifferent toward Home Improvement World and its floor and the little yarn I had to spin for the greater good. She prattled on, "Somebody had to clean it up." I reminded her of depression verging on death, and the distraction I was able to provide with imagery of me pissing on the floor at Home Improvement World. As if that counted for nothing, she repeated, "Somebody had to clean it up."

I reminded her that I was pushed beyond the limits of polite society and its appropriate standards. She repeated the cold, hard fact. I suggested that a bathroom janitor has to deal with worse. But she waited for contrition, so I conceded, short of telling her the truth. "Okay. I'll go and say that I'm sorry and offer to clean the bathrooms."

She granted reprieve. "No. Just, please, don't do that again."

I could have reminded her that Home Improvement World sits on what was recently a lovely field fronting a woodland. But I didn't—and I didn't unravel the yarn, because a good story had worked its magic and we survived, adapting to more or less.

The cats surrounded her every night, each stretching a paw to touch her. They missed her, or maybe they were on assignment. I wanted to get them social security numbers and take the five-hundred-dollar deduction on children. Stella, our youngest, presented her with small snakes. Rachel coddled them, easing them from their fearful coils if necessary. She talked goo goo to them on her way out to the garden, where she released them with everyone's beliefs intact.

I thought about the team for a long time—good people under pressure, often traumatic pressure. But the team huddled by itself, excluding the ball, who was us. You may lose identity on the playing field. You may become an object to be pushed up the field, and the football analogy works. I thought the team needed emotional detachment to better pursue its valiant effort, and that was fine, but the team also needed secrecy to protect itself.

Worse yet, the team presumed idiocy in the patient and the patient's family, who were not pigskins. The team was wrong in its headstrong insistence on correct beliefs.

The legal system requires the team's wily ways. Take Rachel and me, shacked up for years before we were married. Marriage was a formality for us, a social convention. Yet had we been unmarried, we would have been denied communication. Without the social, legal credential, I would have been unqualified to stand guard in the interests of my mate, not allowed on the playing field and hardly the object of the team's appeal to take over for this demented, irrational woman. Without me as legal spouse, Rachel would have been cut and dried, and maybe she'd have done all right.

The team came on strong, assuming that strength necessary to beat the odds. But with no referee to oversee fair interests in comfort and dignity—without someone to blow the whistle in soulful terms, the odds can go longer still. Even if you grant the team the benefit of all doubt, the team may want to frenzy, as seen on TV. Worst of all is the statistical directive of the team. That is, all decision is bound to data-based protocol. Decision defaults to the double blind standard based on the scientific method of theory, experiment, data and conclusion.

Any theory not proven to within the acceptable margin of error, which is four percent, is deemed wrong.

All anecdotal evidence or strong personal belief is deemed wrong. Only those decisions based on the scientific method are defensible in court.

I pondered my behavior and rationale. I considered my overbearing nature. I discounted wrongness and rightness and assessed myself in terms of the difference I made. I factor with consequence at a few junctures. My initial insistence on visiting the corner clinic proved critical. The fundamental importance of that visit to Rachel's survival was the key difference.

Conflict characterized our hospital time. The threat of the condition was made worse by authoritarian dominance and our resistance to it. Most of the turmoil was avoidable with rational dialogue on the front end. Our belief system is based in part on modern medical system error. Horror stories feed prejudice that can only be calmed by calm discourse willing to recognize opinions outside the AMA.

But the AMA paradigm may be changing with the leadership of a few open-minded practitioners who remain mindful that alternate cure can occur, even if only anecdotal. The system changes too with public pressure.

What would we change? We felt segregated from the process. Many people insisted on a nine-inch cut with a scalp peel for removal of a two-inch skull plug so the left temporal lobe of the brain could be lifted, so the clot could be swabbed and the bubble clipped. Close it up, over and out. Yet we got no explanation and disclosure on alternatives or lack thereof. I suspect that the declaration of no alternative was purposefully withheld, on account of potential litigation. Maybe they have a treatment in Podunk Holler, calling for three lizard teeth, a salamander tail and some hind tit pig milk—a recipe that made Old Clem's aneurdiddle flat fucking go away!

But the system cannot share that anecdotal success, since a patient could choose that route and die, and then sue the system. That wouldn't make sense, but the same lawyers who screwed up the system would screw you up again if you try to work around the mess they've made.

But surely some clear and present language could factor the Old-Clem remedy in a practical truth in, say, half a minute or so.

Anxiety is counter-productive. I still feel correct in declining the medivac helicopter, if not for the pressure, then surely for the trauma. The assault would have begun sooner. She would have felt alone and defenseless.

I think postponement of the final angiogram scheduled for ten hours after surgery may have been critical. I think they could have killed her without looking into her eyes or sharing a few words. I think they placed faith solely on the digital readout.

I think Rachel could still be waiting removal from Intensive Care without my insistence on some service around here.

And I suppose all the noise we made resulted in Lawrence of Neurology at the helm. In a system so overwhelmed by legality, rights and representations, the problematic cases gain attention and warrant the best technicians.

But this subject is now polemical.

We got the beer, by the way, hardly green and two months late, but oh, so good. I had three pints, an Irish Blonde, a McCaffrey's Cream Stout and a Harp's on tap. I made acquaintance as well with a Mr. Paddy Jameson, who made perfect sense in a most mellifluous brogue.

Rachel nursed a mango iced tea; she was so reasonable, deferring to Lawrence of Neurology, who proved adept in the other skills, besides those of the invasive technician.

"Oh, gee, you're looking great," he said. He smiled freely at last as he felt the dents and curvature, checking for skull symmetry, left to right, feeling the muscles that were severed just around the corner from the eyebrow, feeling the jaw and nodding in approval. "This aneurysm is gone," he pronounced with vivid finality. Furthermore, "You may resume all of your old activities. You can strain and lift and work out. You can do anything you used to do."

We shared a bright and happy moment, and Rachel said she wanted to be sure he understood her gratitude. Because she *was* grateful, and she wasn't sure that had come across yet. Lawrence said he understood fully; she should not worry about what came across, because she was very confused.

He turned to the movement in his periphery, which was my eyebrow arching. But it settled back down quickly, and I smiled. I didn't remind him that her confusion came from the avalanche rolling down *his* mountain. Because I didn't need to, because some beliefs will not be understood by others. But I was grateful.

"Uh, Doctor, I have a question. We like to travel. Some people might frown on this, but we like to visit, for example, Mexico, and drink tequila. We like to . . . smoke hash in Amsterdam. Do we have any constraints here?"

"No. None. You can do anything you like. But . . . you may observe a more acute sensitivity."

Acute sensitivity is another story. For the time, a civilly cordial exchange was enjoyed by all. I did slip on the way out when the receptionist wanted my parking ticket for validation, "Don't I need psychiatry for that?"

She laughed, "No. I'll make you real." She stamped my ticket, and out we went, into the world of the breathing, joking, living life.

"Where was their sense of humor when we needed it?" I asked. But Rachel was lost in the clouds, drifting happily over the trees. Our cordiality lasted into twilight, in a happy hour of note that started two months late.

Here is what we spent, on our way to clicking our mugs with the Irish, starting out one memorable morning in March:

Physicians' Services (the team)

Intracranial Doppler Stud	$149.00
Twist Drill Implant Rec D	$1,571.00
Craniec Intracranial Aneu	$6,663.00
Use of Operating Microsco	$614.00
Intracranial Doppler Stud	$149.00
Intracranial Doppler Stud	$149.00
Intracranial Doppler Stud	$149.00
Craniect Evac Hemat Intra	$2,571.00
TOTAL	$12,015.00

Hospital Services

Daily Service: 1 Day @ 704.	$704.00
Daily Service: 7 Days @ 2,200.	$15,400.00
Pharmacy	$2,815.57
Med-Surg Supplies	$14,107.28
Laboratory	$1,773.50
Pathology Lab	$83.00
DX X-Ray	$4,250.75
Nuclear Medicine	$1,573.00
CT Scan	$2,860.00
OR Services	$11,615.20
Anesthesia	$1,517.25
Blood Stor-Proc	$468.00
Respiratory SVC	$12.00
Occupation Therp	$86.00
Speech Pathol	$127.25
Emerg Room	$612.50
Pulmonary Func	$26.75
Recovery Room	$878.00
Other DX SVS	$66.50
Other Vascular Studies	$3,129.00
TOTAL	$62,106.05

Bringing the total outlay for the team and the arena to $78,121.05. Add ninety bucks for the very first guy, Bill Varne, who insisted on a pit stop for a CAT scan. It's still very fair, considering the ferry was only $3.75 and the medivac helicopter and limo service would have run another $8,500. The insurance covered eighty percent, so we went out-of-pocket only sixteen grand or so, which is a bargain any day, if you don't count the inconvenience.

We were also gratified that speet patorogy was a pittance at $127.25. We declined the speet patorogy, so we can only presume that the $127.25 was for the consultation. Occupation Therp was also amusing—and a steal at only $86.00. I'm still not clear on what the therapy was, but I'm certain Rachel was rendered more functional. Moreover, you can't get hung up on a few bucks here or there; a month out we got another invoice for $8,205.76 for "additional services," putting us just over eighty-six grand, plus a few bucks for the parking, beer and so on.

Of course I quibbled, but isn't that another certain improvement over judging and insisting?

Life is good. Rachel doesn't drink, because acute sensitivity was putting it politely and is apparently common to post aneurysm people. Best of all, a return to Hawaii and the teeming reefs there and in Fiji, Australia, Palau, Cuba, the Virgins and Philippines with a few more seasons yet to go.